HIGH BLOOD PRESSURE

REVERSAL SECRETS

By

Igor Klibanov

Igor Klibanov

CONTENTS

How you can lower your blood pressure even if it runs in your family... why you don't have to lose weight to lower your blood pressure... why high blood pressure does NOT come with age... a brain problem commonly misdiagnosed as high blood pressure, and how to figure out if you have it

How much does cardio lower your blood pressure?... how many workouts does it take before you see blood pressure reductions (the answer may surprise you)... what's the least amount of cardio you can do, and still lower your blood pressure?... the 3 mechanisms by which cardio lowers your blood pressure... how much does strength training lower your blood pressure?... a simple, little-known 8-minute exercise that lowers your blood pressure by as much as 15.3/7.8... what happens when you combine cardio and strength training... when exercise does NOT lower blood pressure... 2 tests you MUST run before starting a vigorous exercise program (ignore them at your own risk)

The 5 reasons you might have high blood pressure, and the foods that address each reason... the caffeine controversy – settled. Should you stop the caffeine, or keep taking it?... the differences in blood pressure between coffee, green tea, and black tea... which foods to eat less of... alcohol: how much is too much?... hidden food sensitivities that may be raising your blood pressure without you knowing

Two myths about supplements... 3 reasons why I really like supplements... the scientific way to find the right supplement dose... 8 effective supplements, and their dosages... 4 ineffective supplements commonly sold to help lower blood pressure... 3 unproven supplements... how to combine supplements

How short sleep affects your blood pressure... 3 reasons why not getting enough sleep is raising your blood pressure... the prevalence of sleep apnea in the general population vs. in people with high blood pressure... how you can lower your blood pressure by 7.8/5.3 by simply treating undiagnosed sleep apnea... the 8 important basics of sleep hygiene... 3 supplements for sleep

5 important metrics to track to get a handle on your blood pressure... the scientific method of lowering your blood pressure... the fast method of lowering your blood

pressure... the hybrid method of lowering your blood pressure

How the high blood pressure was affecting George... what we learned about George during his initial assessment that allowed us to craft his blood pressure reduction program... what George has tried in the past to help him lower his blood pressure... a week-by-week breakdown of the strategies that we used to drop George's blood pressure... a simple exercise we gave him to do while he was waiting for his doctor to approve his program... a common drink that George was consuming that kept his blood pressure elevated... the foods that George ate that lowered his blood pressure... the exercise strategies that George used... the magnesium dose that George used to lower his high blood pressure... 4 things that could have gone even better, and lowered his high blood pressure even more

Acknowledgements

In this section, I would like to acknowledge and thank the people without whom this book would have been complete, unintelligible gibberish. These people helped with editing, making the text easy-to-read, and suggested which illustrations to include. In no particular order:

Roni Shae is the illustrator for this book. He's a talented high school student, with a bright future in design.

George Stavrou is both a friend and former client who has decades of experience in the fitness/nutrition industry, and now, runs a comprehensive online health program called "The Stavrou Method." You can check it out by visiting https://thestavroumethod.com

Dr. Romi Fung is a Naturopathic Physician in Richmond, British Columbia. He has extensive knowledge in mental health and has clinical interests in treating Alzheimer's Disease and Dementia

Riaz Aziz is a colleague, strength & nutrition coach, and Cancer Recovery Specialist. As a cancer survivor with a busy family life, and business he graciously carved out some time to assist with editing this book. To enlist his services as a Cancer Recovery Specialist, visit www.ibeatcancernowwhat.com

Shaneh-Abbas Jaffer has worked with Fitness Solutions Plus for over 4 years at the time of this writing. He was one of the founders of the FSP online training program. He is a Registered Kinesiolgist and Nurse. Check his articles out on chronic injuries/illness and more at www.myofiber.ca

Jo Morgan Dakin is a follower of my posts who is controlling her high blood pressure through my tips and knows where a sentence ends and where a comma should be used.

Jenny Teplitsky who is a former client, long-time friend and reader. She is an Engineer who loves learning about fitness and nutrition.

Introduction

You're probably holding this book because either you have high blood pressure, or your stubborn husband/wife/mother/father has it. You/they might have just gotten the diagnosis recently, or maybe you've had it for years (or even decades). And you've gone to Dr. Google to see the consequences of it:

- Heart attack

- Stroke

- Aneurysm

- Memory problems

    ...and other things you don't want to get.

Then you start imagining your future if you have one of those (and survive). You would:

- Not be able to do the things you love, whether it's gardening, playing golf, travelling, playing with your kids or grandkids, etc.

- Have to visit the doctor way more often than you do now

- Be a burden on your family members

But fortunately, it doesn't have to be that way. These consequences are anything but inevitable. The fact that you're holding this book (or reading it on your screen) means that you won't go down without a fight.

And you, my friend, are the kind of person who will greatly benefit from this book.

Each chapter is a stand-alone chapter. In other words, you don't need to read the previous chapters to benefit from the advice in any individual chapter.

What Can You Expect?

You might be wondering a few things:

- What do I have to do to lower my blood pressure naturally?

- Do I have to give up the foods I love?

- Does supplement work?

- Will I need to spend hours and hours every week at the gym?

   …and the big one: do I have to lose weight to lower my blood pressure?

To answer your questions:

What you have to do to lower your blood pressure: follow the advice in this book. Either just the bits and pieces that are easy for you to do, or the whole thing. Of course, you'll get the greatest, fastest and most long-lasting reductions if you follow everything. But even if you can't or don't want to, that's fine. Any single strategy here can reduce your blood pressure. And every little bit counts. In fact, small reductions in blood pressure can result in very large improvements in health, even if your blood pressure is still above normal.

Do you have to give up the foods you love? Although it might be helpful, you'll learn about some foods that you can include that will lower your blood pressure even without giving up the foods you love. After all, it's much easier to add foods to your diet, than to remove them.

Do supplements work? The only thing I can guarantee is this: nothing works for 100% of the people, 100% of the time. Not medications, not surgery, not exercise, not supplements. However, I will tell you about several supplements that have the most potent effects on your blood pressure, with minimal-to-no side effects. And I'll also tell you which supplements are not worth your money.

Will you need to spend hours and hours each week at the gym? You can if you want to. But I'll show you an 8-minute exercise that you can do at home, without any equipment and reduce your blood pressure as well as hours on the treadmill.

Will you need to lose weight to lower your blood pressure? If you're overweight, losing weight may benefit your health. But with the strategies in this book, you'll be able to lower your blood pressure, even without losing weight.

Sounds like a good deal? Good. I want you to succeed at this.

This book is aimed to satisfy both the geek, who wants to know the mechanisms, and the science behind all the recommendations, as well as the "give me the bottom line" straight shooter.

Want the bottom line without any of the science? Flip to the conclusion chapter, and you'll find your high blood pressure program in an accessible spot, where you can consume it in under 5 minutes – without the scientific explanations.

About the Author

And hey, if we're going to spend the next few hours together, why don't we get better acquainted?

Let me introduce myself.

I'm Igor. Nice to meet ya…..

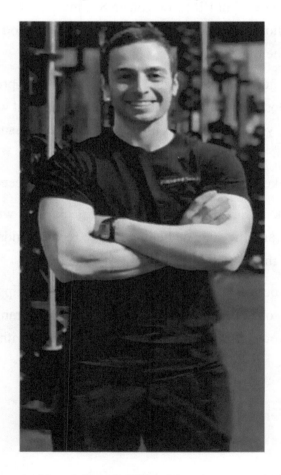

I have a degree in kinesiology and health science, as well as multiple diplomas in clinical nutrition. I was selected as one of the top 5 personal trainers in Toronto by the Metro News newspaper, written 5 other books besides this one, as well as over 450 articles (at the time of this writing) on my blog (FitnessSolutionsPlus.ca/blog). I've been hired by some of Canada's largest corporations to speak on the topics of how to reverse chronic conditions, and have done approximately 50 speaking engagements per year for the last 9 years.

So, you might ask "why is a personal trainer writing about high blood pressure?" Because unlike most personal trainers, who work with athletes, models and bodybuilders, my specialty is "the big 4 plus 1."

The big 4, being:

- High blood pressure

- Type 2 diabetes

- Arthritis

- Osteoporosis

The "plus 1" is menopause.

People seek us out not when they want bigger biceps, but when they don't want to go on medications for the rest of their life.

Because of that, I spent a lot time and money researching the best, most effective ways to lower blood pressure, from 3 perspectives:

- Exercise

- Nutrition

- Supplements

I even created a certification that teaches other personal trainers how to do the same thing. That certification is called the "Top 1% Trainer Program." If you're a fitness professional, and want to get certified, just visit https://www.FitnessSolutionsPlus.ca/top-1-percent-2. If you'd like a special, $300 discount on it, just email me at Igor@TorontoFitnessOnline.com.

The same goes for you, my dear reader. I LOOOOOVVVEEEE hearing success stories. I want to hear yours. So after you've lowered your own blood pressure, I want to hear from you. Email me, and let me know how you did.

4 Common Myths About High Blood Pressure

There are plenty of myths around high blood pressure. Some of them, you might actually believe. Lucky for you that you're reading this book, because in this chapter, we'll bust 4 of the most common myths about high blood pressure.

In no particular order:

Myth #1: It Runs in My Family, So There's Nothing I Can Do About It

Not true. What a lot of people blame on "genetics" is really just **inherited environment**. If your eating, exercise, and sleep patterns are the same as your parents and grandparents, you'll get the conditions that they got.

There's a saying that "**genetics load the gun, but environment pulls the trigger**." That is to say that you may have the genes for high blood pressure, but **genes are not destiny**. Rather, they're more like an on/off switch. If the environment is right, the switch will be turned on (you'll get high blood pressure). If the environment is not conducive to high blood pressure (and therefore, conducive to good health), the switch will be turned off.

So yes, your whole family may have high blood pressure, but you don't have to get it as well. Or, if you already have it, in a very large number of cases, it's highly reversible. Follow the advice in this book for at least a month, and see if that doesn't turn it around.

Myth #2: You Have to Lose Weight to Lower Your Blood Pressure

This one makes perfect sense. After all, the theory goes, if you have too much body fat, it compresses arteries, and raises blood pressure, or the heart must supply blood to a larger body, so it has to pump harder.

But there's a mountain of studies (many of them included in the different chapters throughout this book) showing decreased blood pressure when X increases/decreases (where "X" can be potassium, magnesium, sodium, etc.), without concurrent decreases in weight.

So maybe it's not the weight loss that's causing the lower blood pressure, but the stuff you have to do to lose weight, like eat a diet higher in vegetables (higher potassium and magnesium), and lower in processed food (therefore lower in sodium). But what if calories were the same, but potassium and magnesium increased, and sodium decreased? Or what if your weight stayed the same, but you started exercising? Or what if your weight stayed the same, but you took a supplement to help you lower blood pressure? Would it work? The research is fairly conclusive on this one: yes!

That's not to say that you shouldn't lose weight if you've got the weight to lose. It will have other benefits besides lowering blood pressure. But as anyone who's ever tried to lose weight knows, it's a long, slow, laborious process. Losing 50 pounds might take 25-75 weeks. **But normalizing blood pressure? That can be done in a month or less** (see chapter 6 on how to do that).

In fact, with many of my clients, their blood pressure normalizes far before their weight comes into the "ideal" range.

Myth #3: High Blood Pressure Just Comes with Age

Not true. If age was the single most important factor in the development of high blood pressure, then everyone over a certain age would have it. But not everyone does.

There's a saying that **"time amplifies bad habits."** If you have a bad habit for a year, that's not great. But if you carry the same bad habit for 40 years, well, it's a lot worse, and you'll feel the consequences much more.

You don't exercise when you're 25? No big deal (not great, but the effects aren't noticeable yet). You don't exercise when you're 65? Big deal.

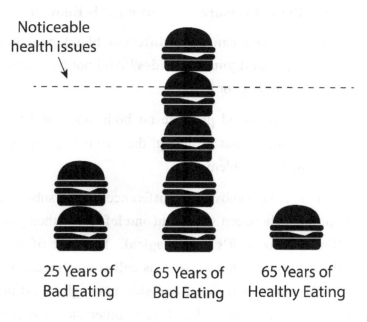

Noticeable
health issues

25 Years of
Bad Eating

65 Years of
Bad Eating

65 Years of
Healthy Eating

You eat poorly when you're 25? No big deal. You eat poorly when you're 65? That's 40 more years than 25 years of bad eating.

So it's not like high blood pressure just comes with age – it doesn't. **Your bad habits have greater consequences the longer you've been doing them**.

Fortunately, many of these bad consequences are reversible. You have high blood pressure? That's because you're sending signals to the body, to make it believe like high blood pressure is advantageous to the inputs you're putting in. Change the inputs (exercise, nutrition, supplements, sleep), and your output changes (lower blood pressure, more energy, less body fat, better sleep, etc.).

Myth #4: One Blood Pressure Measurement is Enough

Did you know that **you can have different blood pressure readings between your right and your left sides**? And not by a little bit, either, but as much as 15 mmHg, or more.

If you have high blood pressure on both sides, and the difference between sides is only about 5 mmHg, then your high blood pressure is truly a cardiovascular problem.

But if you do have a substantial difference (again, substantial is about 15 mmHg or more) between your right and left sides, then **your problem isn't cardiovascular – it's neurological.** The part of the brain that controls blood pressure on both sides is called the "medulla oblongata", which is in the brain stem. So if one side has high blood pressure, it's important to test the other side. If your other side has normal blood pressure, then the treatment should be neurologically-oriented. Not aimed towards the heart.

There's a decent number of people out th
inappropriately being treated for high blood pre
problem is with the brain stem.

Now that we've busted some of the most common
blood pressure, let's talk about what to actually do to reverse it.

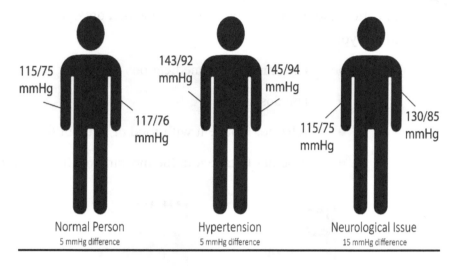

The Exercise Prescription for Lower Blood Pressure

Y ou know how when you go to your doctor and s/he prescribes a medication, there's a lot of precision behind that prescription? Your doctor will tell you:

- The name of the medication

- The dosage

- Whether to take it with food or without food

- Whether to take it in the morning or the evening

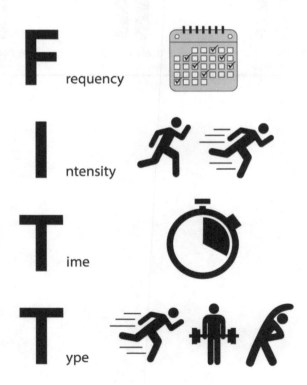

F requency

I ntensity

T ime

T ype

And yet, when your doctor recommends exercise, they just leave it at that: "you should exercise. It's good for you." But no more details than that. You have to guess important details, like:

- Should you do cardio, strength training or stretching?

- How many days per week?

- At what intensity (heart rate, perceived exertion, or percentage of your maximum weight)?

- For what duration?

...and more.

Just as a doctor would not prescribe the same medication for different conditions, nor does it make sense to do the same type of exercise for different conditions. What's good for one can be bad for another. Hence the need for precision in exercise prescription.

This chapter will give you that precision, whether you're a lay person, a medical professional, or a fitness professional.

This chapter will cover:

- The effects of cardio

- The mechanisms behind how cardio lowers blood pressure

- The effects of strength training.

- The mechanisms behind strength training's anti-hypertensive effects

- The effects of combining cardio with strength training. Do they add to each other's effects? Or cancel them out?

- When exercise does not work. Nothing works 100% of the time, for 100% of people, so it's important to identify for whom exercise will not be effective.

- Bottom line: key exercise recommendations and takeaways.

Ready? Let's get started.

The Effects of Cardio on Blood Pressure

There has been a lot of research done on how cardio affects blood pressure, all meant to answer different questions.

A 2002 clinical trial[1] on blood pressure reduction in mature patients wanted to answer the question of "to what extent can cardio lower blood pressure in the elderly who have high blood pressure?"

They found that **a single workout lowers blood pressure** by between 5-7 mmHg. If your regular blood pressure is 140/90, a single workout can lower it down as low as 133/83. Not bad. And the effects last for 24 hours afterwards.

This drop in blood pressure after exercise is called "**post exercise hypotension**" (or PEH for short).

A study by leading scientists[2] on exercise and ambulatory blood pressure wanted to compare the effects of **steady training (where you maintain the same pace for 20+ minutes) against interval training** (where you go fast for 30 seconds to 3 minutes, and then, you go slow for that same period of time). In both cases, the results slightly favoured steady state training. In the group that did steady state, both their systolic and diastolic blood pressure fell by 4-8 mmHg. The group that did interval training had a drop of 5-6 mmHg, but only in the diastolic blood pressure.

If all this talk of "systolic" and "diastolic" blood pressure means nothing to you, let me explain (or just check out the diagram below). You know how when you get your blood pressure reading, it says (for example) 120/80? The top number (120) is your systolic blood pressure. And the bottom number (80) is your diastolic blood pressure. Your systolic blood pressure is how much pressure your blood exerts against the arteries when your heart contracts. Your diastolic blood pressure is how much pressure your blood exerts against the arteries when your heart relaxes. Capisce?

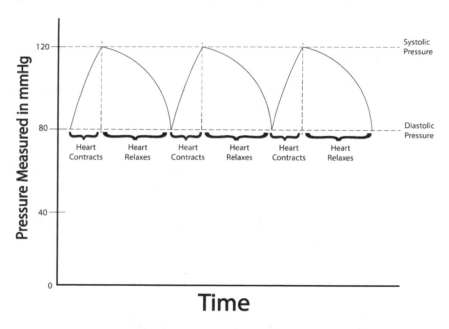

Recently, some scientists comparing exercise intensity and hypotension[3] wanted to answer the question of optimal intensity. **Is there an optimal intensity at which to exercise to lower blood pressure**? Is it a "more is better" type of thing, or is there a point which is optimal? The short answer: it seems that yes, in this case, more is better. Here's what they did:

They took 45 middle-aged, overweight men with blood pressures ranging from 120/80 (the average was 144.5/84.4 mmHg), up to 159/99, and poor cholesterol profiles. They were divided into 4 groups:

Group 1 did nothing. They were the control group

Group 2 exercised at 40% of their maximal aerobic capacity

Group 3 exercised at 60% of their maximal aerobic capacity

Group 4 went all out, and exercised at 100% of their maximal capacity

The results were:

- Group 2 reduced their systolic blood pressure by an average of 2.8 mmHg, and their diastolic blood pressure by 1.5 mmHg.

- Group 3 reduced their systolic blood pressure by an average of 5.4 mmHg, and their diastolic by 2.0 mmHg.

- Group 4 reduced their systolic blood pressure by an average of 11.7 mmHg, and their diastolic by 4.9 mmHg.

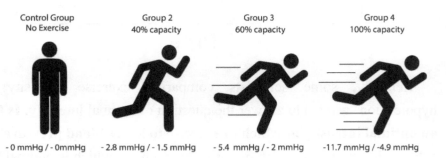

Control Group No Exercise	Group 2 40% capacity	Group 3 60% capacity	Group 4 100% capacity
- 0 mmHg / - 0mmHg	- 2.8 mmHg / - 1.5 mmHg	- 5.4 mmHg / - 2 mmHg	-11.7 mmHg / -4.9 mmHg

And a study by leading sports scientists [4] wanted to answer the question of **whether there was a difference between the effects of a single workout, and long-term training**. The short answer: there isn't. With aerobic exercise (cardio), if you stop exercising, your blood pressure rises back up. The verdict is: just like with medications: if you stop taking them, blood pressure rises, the same happens with cardio. You stop doing your cardio, your blood pressure rises as well.

This, however is in contrast to strength training. With strength training, any drops in blood pressure are actually maintained once you stop working out. Not forever, but for a few weeks, up to a few months. We'll talk about that in greater detail later.

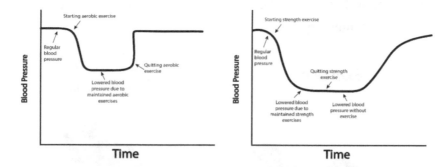

The final piece of the puzzle is duration. **What's the least amount of time that you need to exercise to lower your blood pressure?**

A study published recently[5] on the influence of dynamic exercise on blood pressure decided to investigate that.

The researchers took 45 men with high blood pressure (average of 144.6/85.2), and divided them into 5 groups:

Group 1 was the control group. They didn't exercise.

Group 2 exercised for 15 minutes at a low intensity (40%)

ρ 3 exercised for 15 minutes at a moderate intensity (60%)

ıup 4 exercised for 30 minutes at a low intensity (40%)

Group 5 exercised for 30 minutes at a moderate intensity (60%)

Even with only 15 minutes of exercise and a low intensity, group 2 lowered their systolic blood pressure by 5.6 mmHg (which is almost 19% of the excess blood pressure). Diastolic blood pressure was reduced by 2.1 mmHg (which is almost 21% of the excess blood pressure).

There are of course greater reductions with greater durations and greater intensities, but this previous study didn't look at "what's optimum?" Rather, they looked at "what's minimum? **What's the least you can do, and still get a benefit**?" And the answer is "just 15 minutes, at a fairly low intensity."

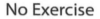

No Exercise

15 minutes
40% intensity

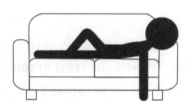

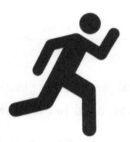

- 0 mmHg / - 0mmHg

- 5.6 mmHg / - 2.1 mmHg
-19% excess / -21% excess

The answer to "what's optimum" is much more complicated than "what's the minimum?" And unfortunately, that answer doesn't exist yet, since there's no universal optimum. What's optimum for men might or might not be different for women (it hasn't been investigated yet). What's optimum might differ based on whether you have prehypertension (blood pressures from 120/80, up to 139/89), or full-out hypertension (higher than 140/90). Or it might not. Again, we don't know. Optimum might differ based on whether someone is taking medications or not taking medications. Or it might not. Once again, we don't know.

So yes, there is still a lot that is unknown about exercise and blood pressure, but in this section, you saw the available information on how different variables affect it.

How Cardio Works to Lower Blood Pressure (The Mechanisms)

In the previous section, we learned that cardio does indeed work to lower blood pressure. If that's good enough for you, and you don't care about the mechanisms, you can skip this section. But if you're my geeky friend, and you want to know, keep reading.

Currently, there are 3 known potential mechanisms by which cardio lowers blood pressure.

Mechanism #1: Increased Arterial Diameter

In someone who has high blood pressure, one layer of the artery, called the "intima media" gets thicker. Like a muscle gets thicker from strength training, so too does this layer of the artery as a result of high blood pressure.

The Structure of an Artery Wall

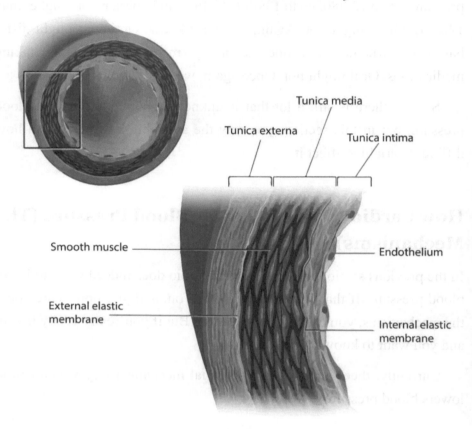

_A group of researchers[6], found that the thickness of the intima media decreases as a result of cardio. As a result of decreased thickness, the diameter increases.

Mechanism #2: Increased Bioavailability of Nitric Oxide

Nitric oxide is a molecule inside the body that helps "open up" blood vessels. We all have it, but those with high blood pressure simply can't use it effectively.

A study published[7] on systemic **alpha-adrenergic** and nitric oxide inhibition on basal limb blood flow in middle age and older individuals, found that aerobic exercise re-sensitizes the cells to nitric oxide, so it can exert its artery-widening effects again.

Mechanism #3: Increased Baroreflex Sensitivity

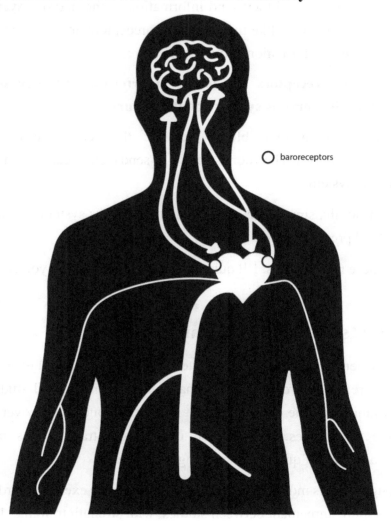

O baroreceptors

Don't let your brain shut off when you read the word "baroreflex." In typical Igor-fashion, I won't leave you hanging there with terminology you don't know.

What is the baroreflex? The nervous system has receptors all over the body that send information back up to the nervous system about different kinds of information. For example, mechanoreceptors are found in muscles and joints, and they send information to the nervous system about mechanical stimuli (like touch). Thermoreceptors are found in the skin, and they send information about temperature.

Likewise, **baroreceptors are found in arteries, and they send information to the nervous system about pressure**.

In someone with high blood pressure, the sensitivity of the baroreceptors decreases. They don't receive or send clear signals from and to the nervous system.

With cardio, the signals are clearer, and the nervous system is able to regulate blood pressure better.

Study these mechanisms. I'll quiz you on them when I see you ;)

The Effects of Strength Training

Typically, when medical professionals tell you that you should exercise, they mostly refer to cardio, so cardio has been extremely well studied. Strength training, on the other hand, not as much. Nonetheless, over the last couple of decades, the research on strength training has been mounting, and a lot of questions are being answered.

Although there is more research available on aerobic exercise (cardio), and there's more agreement between studies, with strength training, there is some conflicting research. Yet, in the studies that show a positive effect on blood pressure from strength training, the **drops are larger than with cardio**.

In 2013,a research team[8], studied a group of elderly people with high blood pressure exercised under 2 different conditions:

- Condition 1: they did strength training with 50% of their maximal weight,

- Condition 2: they exercised at 80% of the maximal weight.

The exercises were identical. When they exercised at 50% of their maximum, their blood pressure was reduced by 23/7 mmHg (down from 147/93 mmHg). But **at 80%, their blood pressure was reduced by 33/15** (down from 148/90 mmHg).

50% maximal weight   80% maximal weight

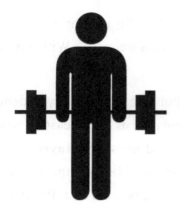   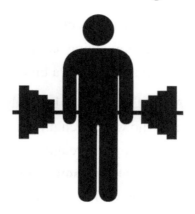

- 23 mmHg / - 7mmHg   - 33 mmHg / - 15 mmHg

If you're reading this, and thinking "I have to test my maximal weight", don't. Not unless you're doing it under professional supervision (if they think it's a good idea). For your purposes, a general guideline is that at 80% of your maximal weight, you can do around 10 reps (give or take two) before you can't do any more. At 50% of your maximal weight, you might be about to do 25-30 reps.

Traditionally, it has been recommended that people with high blood pressure avoid very heavy weights, because heavier weights raise blood pressure too high. And that is true. However, after the end of the exercise, blood pressure returns to normal within about 10 seconds. This has been most advice to stay on the safe side, "just in case", but really, we don't know how risky heavy weights are for people with high blood pressure. In this study, heavy weights were more beneficial than light weights, but keep in mind, that the participants were exercising under medical supervision. Until further research is available on the risk-to-benefit ratio of heavy weights in people with high blood pressure, I'd advise the same thing: don't do it. How heavy is heavy? If you can't do it more than 5 times, it's heavy.

We know that with cardio, the effects of cardio last for only about a day. You stop doing cardio, and blood pressure rises. With strength training, it seems to be a bit different.

According to a 2014 study[9] it was found that in elderly sedentary women who were strength training on a regular basis for at least 14 weeks, and then stopped strength training, their **blood pressure stayed low for up to 14 weeks without exercise**. What happened beyond the 14 weeks? We don't know. The researchers didn't measure beyond that. But it's nice to know that even if you miss a few days, your blood pressure won't shoot back up.

Here's another cool effect of strength training: according to some studies (like research on resistance training and blood pressure[10] and studies undertaken on strength training and haemodynamic response[11]), even in the cases when strength training doesn't decrease blood pressure at rest, **it does minimize the rise in blood pressure during cardio**.

Lately, a little bit of research has been coming out on the very impressive effects of **static strength training** on blood pressure. What's the difference between static strength training, and dynamic strength training? Dynamic strength training (AKA isotonic strength training) is the stuff you usually see at the gym, and most of the exercises that you think of, like squats, deadlifts, bench press, overhead press, etc. Static strength training (AKA isometrics) is when you hold a position, or squeeze a muscle.

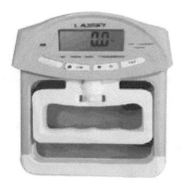

Hand Grip Dynamometer

As it's done in research, scientists make the participants squeeze a device called a "hand grip dynamometer."

They do it for 4 sets of 2 minutes, at 30% of their maximum, resting 3 minutes between sets, and they do this 3 times per week. That's only 8 minutes of "exercise", 3 times per week.

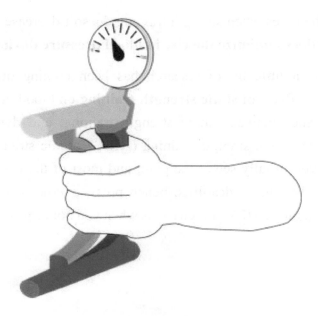

Although the research on static strength training (specifically, grip training) is in its infancy, the results are promising. One meta-analysis conducted in 2010[12] , found reductions of 15.3/7.8 mmHg. Better than the effects seen with cardio, and it only takes 8 minutes per day, 3 times per week. Almost sounds like an infomercial, but this is what the current available research is showing.

Again, it's still in its infancy, and much more research is necessary, but **for a very small time investment, the payoff in results can be very impressive**.

Although research on strength training is growing, there is still not much information to answer the questions of "what's the optimal frequency?", "what's the minimal frequency?", "what's the optimal intensity?", "what's the minimal intensity?", and others.

At best, we can say that we know strength training is good, but we don't yet know the optimal protocols, or the smallest "dose" necessary to have an effect.

How Does Strength Training Work?

As mentioned earlier, not as much is known about strength training as about cardio in relation to high blood pressure, but from the little we do know, the primary mechanism by which strength training reduces blood pressure is also through **reduced thickness of the artery wall**, according to clinical trials on artery adaptations published recently[13].

There are likely other mechanisms at work, but we're not yet sure what they are. After all, what is it about strength training that makes the effects last when someone takes a 14-week break from it, but with cardio the effects are gone after 1 day? There has to be more at play.

The Effects of Concurrent Training: Do You Get Better Effects When Combining Strength Training with Cardio?

We know that cardio lowers blood pressure, and strength training also lowers blood pressure. So in theory, you would think that combining cardio and strength training would lower blood pressure more. After all, 1+1= 2. Right? Well, that's actually not so clear, and the research on that is pretty mixed.

The research, however, is clear on one thing: there is no additive effect. At best, doing concurrent training is no better than doing either cardio or strength training by itself. At worst, the effects of cardio and strength training cancel each other out, and there's no effect on blood pressure whatsoever.

In one study on acute and chronic cardiovascular responses[14], the researchers had hypertensive older women, who were taking medications for their blood pressure perform both strength training and cardio in the same workout. The results were disappointing. Average blood pressure dropped by about 3-5 mmHg. Both cardio and strength training by themselves have stronger effects.

Unfortunately, there are no studies showing that blood pressure drops are better with concurrent training than with either cardio or strength training in isolation.

The inquisitive folks might be wondering "why?" Why are there no additive effects when you combine cardio with strength training? Unfortunately, the research doesn't really try to answer that question, so I'll give my opinion.

I think that one possible mechanism is the "ceiling effect." That is, after blood pressure has already dropped a substantial amount, and gotten close to normal, it may be hard (and unnecessary) to drop it even lower.

Interestingly enough, though there is evidence[14] that shows that order matters. **Should you do cardio before strength training, or strength training before cardio?** According to the previous study, doing cardio after strength training results in larger drops in blood pressure, compared to strength training after cardio. Cool, eh?

When Exercise Does Not Work to Lower Blood Pressure

We wish that exercise worked for everyone all the time, but unfortunately nothing works for 100% of the people, 100% of the time. Not medications, not surgery, and not exercise.

Therefore, it's important to know when exercise does not work.

First of all, **exercise fails to lower blood pressure about 20-25% of the time.** That doesn't mean it doesn't have other benefits. It'll make you stronger, give you more endurance, have positive effects on other systems of your body (your nervous system, endocrine system, immune system, etc.). It just won't affect your blood pressure.

Fortunately, you know very quickly whether you're a "non-responder." Given that drops in blood pressure are seen in a matter of hours after exercise, and they're the same for first-time exercisers as well as experienced exercisers, **if after the first session, your blood pressure doesn't drop in a matter of a few hours, you might be a non-responder to exercise** (again, only as far as blood pressure is concerned. It'll have other positive effects outside of blood pressure).

Some very preliminary research[15] suggests that the **non-responders likely have high CRP and fibrinogen levels** (these are both markers of inflammation) in addition to their high blood pressure. This may be tied to high stress levels and/or poor sleep. However, those with high blood sugar levels, and a poor cholesterol profile do respond very well to exercise.

Again, I want to emphasize that this doesn't mean that if your blood pressure doesn't change in response to exercise that it means that exercise is useless. It just means that it doesn't affect your blood pressure, but it will positively affect a lot of other things, like your strength, energy levels, mobility, and more.

Safety Precautions Before Exercise (Neglect These at Your Own Risk)

You've now read all about the benefits of exercise, and are excited by the blood pressure-lowering potential of it. You can't wait to jump in.

But I'd advise you to wait. Don't start exercising yet. If you haven't exercised in a long time (that's 6 months or longer), the American Heart Association, in its position statement[16], titled *"Placing the Risks Into Perspective: A Scientific Statement From the American Heart Association Council on Nutrition, Physical Activity, and Metabolism and the Council on Clinical Cardiology"*, recommends testing before you jump into a vigorous exercise program (anything over 70% of your maximal heart rate).

They recommend doing 2 tests to clear you for exercise:

1. The cardiac stress test

2. Atherosclerotic risk profile

Speak to your doctor about running these two tests to see if the benefits of vigorous exercise outweigh the risks for you. If you already have high blood pressure, and you choose to skip these two tests may expose you to unnecessary risk of a heart attack or stroke – the very things you're trying to avoid.

When NOT to Exercise

Exercise is definitely good for you, but like anything, it carries with it some inherent risks. The healthier you are, the lower your risks.

But there are 2 cases when you should NOT exercise, according to a study on exercise and cardiovascular health[17].

If you wake up one day, and your systolic blood pressure is over 200 mmHg, or your diastolic is above 110 mmHg at rest.

> 1. If during exercise, your blood pressure goes above 250 mmHg for your systolic, and 115 mmHg for your diastolic. Stop your exercise immediately, and seek medical attention.

Bottom Line and Key Takeaways

With all this information, what's the bottom line? What do I recommend?

If you (or your patient) are a regular exerciser, and you've built the habit of exercise, then follow the available evidence:

- Do cardio 3-5 days per week:

  o The intensity should be over 75% of your maximal heart rate (which, theoretically is 220 minus your age. So if you're 60, your maximum is theoretically 160, and 75% of that is 120 beats per minute).

  o Do it for about 30-50 minutes each workout

  o The type doesn't matter, whether you're jogging, or cycling, or swimming, or on the elliptical.

- Do strength training 2-3 times per week:

- o Lift weights heavy enough that you can't do them more than 20 times, but light enough that you can do more than 5 times.

  - o Do 2-5 sets per exercise

  - o Do 8-10 exercises per workout

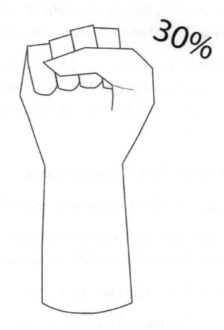

If you (or your patient) are not a regular exerciser, go with the "low-dose, high-effectiveness" training:

- • Squeeze both hands into fists with about 30% of your full force

  - o Hold for 2 minutes per contraction.

  - o Repeat 4 times, resting 3 minutes in between contractions o   Do this 3 times per week

Although this type of training has no proven benefit on your endurance, or other markers of health (like blood sugar, cholesterol, inflammation, etc.), it does work to reduce blood pressure. And doing this is better than doing nothing.

Nutrition for
High Blood Pressure

"You should lose weight and lower your salt intake." That's about the extent of the advice that people get when trying to lower their blood pressure.

While it may be sensible advice, there are a number of other, easy things you can do to lower your blood pressure.

That's what you'll learn about in this chapter:

- The 5 reasons someone might have high blood pressure

- Which foods to eat more of to help you lower your blood pressure

- The caffeine controversy

- Which foods to eat less of

The coolest part is you **don't need to lose weight** to lower your blood pressure. That's not to say that you shouldn't. If you're overweight, losing weight will certainly make you healthier, but it's not a requirement for improving your blood pressure.

5 Reasons for High Blood Pressure

There is more than one reason why blood pressure might be high:

Stress

If you've been reading about health, you must have come across a hormone called "cortisol." The media has dubbed it "the stress hormone."

For good reason. Because your body releases more of it when you're under stress.

See, you release cortisol all the time anyway, whether you're stressed, or relaxed. You just release more of it under stress.

Since our bodies have not caught up to the modern world, they're stuck in a world that's about 40,000 years old. Forty thousand years ago, about **the only 2 things that stressed us out were famines and sabre-toothed tigers**.

Just think about it, if you're running away from a sabre-toothed tiger, you'd want:

- Your blood sugar to rise, to give fuel to working muscles

- Your blood pressure to rise, to push the blood to your legs faster

- Your digestion to stop working, so that it doesn't use up energy that should be getting used up by the muscles

- Your reproductive system to stop working, also to not use up energy that should be getting used up by the muscles

From an evolutionary perspective, **high blood pressure was very beneficial**, because it was just temporary, until the stressor went away. But in our modern world, we're not stressed because we're running away from a sabre-toothed tiger. Instead, we're stressed because of relationships, finances, deadlines, etc. However, to our body, it doesn't matter. **Whether stress is physical (exercise or famine), or mental/emotional, the hormonal response is the same: high cortisol**.

In the pharmaceutical world, the way they deal with it is by blocking adrenaline (which is basically turbo-charged cortisol) either at the level of the heart (the term for that is "beta blockers"), or at the level of the brain (the term for that is "central alpha agonists").

Are there foods that do this naturally? Yep. **Celery (2-3 medium stalks) and garlic (2-3 cloves)**. In fact, one thorough meta-analysis[18] showed that garlic can lower blood pressure by as much as 8.4/7.2 mmHg.

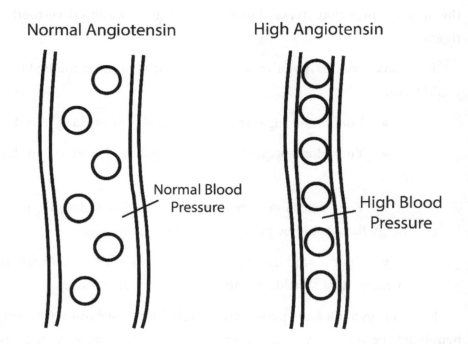

Normal Angiotensin — Normal Blood Pressure

High Angiotensin — High Blood Pressure

Narrow Arteries

Arteries take blood away from the heart. They're a tube. But if that tube gets narrower, the blood will push out against the walls harder. After all, the volume of blood in your body doesn't change. But if there's less space for that blood, it will push out against the arteries harder.

What causes the arteries to narrow? A hormone called **"angiotensin."** That's why in the pharmaceutical world, there's a class of drugs called

"**ACE inhibitors**", which stands for angiotensin-converting-enzyme inhibitors. Without getting too deep into the mechanism of action, the end result is lower angiotensin levels, and therefore, wider blood vessels.

Fortunately, natural compounds found in normal foods can also inhibit this enzyme, and widen blood vessels. What are some examples of foods that open up blood vessels by decreasing angiotensin?

- Dairy products (especially cheddar cheese, gouda, yogurt and sour milk)
- Egg yolks
- Tuna
- Beef
- Sardines
- Garlic
- Spinach
- Grapes
- Broccoli
- Buckwheat
- Rice

Think it makes sense to eat these if you want to lower blood pressure? You bet!

By the way, this list is by no means exhaustive. There was one very comprehensive study done on the subject, so for the geeks who want to delve deeper into it, check it out here; *(https://onlinelibrary.wiley.com/doi/full/10.1111/1541-4337.12051)19*

Another way to make arteries open wider is not to affect angiotensin, but to prevent the muscles surrounding your arteries from contracting. The mineral needed for arteries to contract is calcium. So we want to prevent calcium from binding to its receptors on muscle cells, which causes them to contract. In pharmaceutical terms, these are called "**calcium channel blockers**."

If you're wondering "are there foods that can naturally act as calcium channel blockers?" The answer is yes! **Celery (again, 2-3 medium stalks) and garlic (2-3 cloves)** act as natural calcium channel blockers, according to a study[20] on hypertension, drugs, nutrition and nutraceuticals. If you're wondering "should I avoid calcium supplements?", unfortunately I have to refer you to your pharmacist on that one, since there are a number of different considerations.

Excess Fluid/High Sodium

Another potential reason why blood pressure might be high is due to **excess fluid inside the arteries**. You might be wondering "how does excess fluid end up in the arteries in the first place?" Good question. When you eat more sodium than you should, your body holds on to it. **Sodium attracts water**, so you don't just get sodium, you get more water in the arteries than you should have.

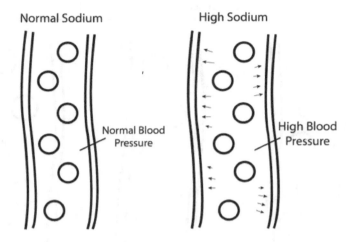

That's why there's a class of drugs known as **"diuretics"** that help the body get rid of excess sodium, and along with it, excess water. Less water in the arteries, less force against the arteries.

Are there foods with natural diuretic properties? You bet! Parsley (minimum half a cup), asparagus (minimum half a cup, or 6 medium spears), watermelon (1 cup), and **celery (2-3 stalks)** all fit the bill (hmm… did we just see celery in 3 different categories? I think we did!).

Low Potassium

The mineral that counterbalances sodium is potassium. When you eat the right amount of potassium (which is around 4700 mg/day), it keeps sodium in balance, which in turn prevents excess water from accumulating inside the arteries. Additionally, **potassium opens up blood vessels in its own right**.

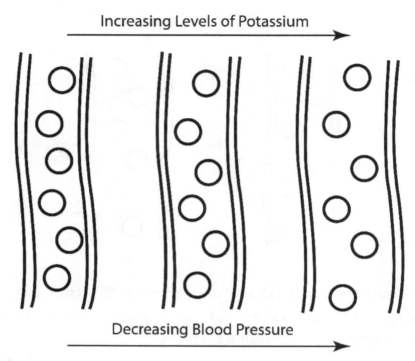

Increasing Levels of Potassium

Decreasing Blood Pressure

In fact, one study[21] found that **the higher the dietary potassium intake, the lower the blood pressure**, and the greatest effects of dietary potassium happen in those with higher blood pressure.

In another study[22] comparing the effects of dietary potassium intake and the need for antihypertensive medication, a group of people was told to increase potassium in their diet (and the researchers measured that indeed, they were consuming more potassium by checking their urine for potassium), and found that **81% of people who increased their potassium intake lowered their medications by 50%. The real cool part is that these changes happened without any loss in weight**.

Which foods are high in potassium?

- Dates (5 dates are about 835 mg of potassium)

- Prunes (10 prunes are nearly 700 mg)

- Potatoes (one large potato has about 1600 mg)

- Bananas (1 medium banana has about 422 mg)

- Avocados (half an avocado has nearly 500 mg)

- Sun-dried tomatoes (20 sun-dried tomatoes have about 1400 mg)

- Sweet potatoes (1 cup of sweet potatoes has about 950 mg)

Low Magnesium

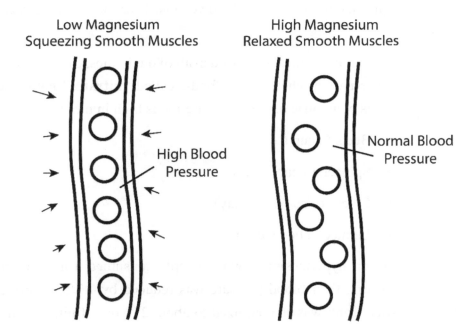

Low Magnesium
Squeezing Smooth Muscles

High Magnesium
Relaxed Smooth Muscles

High Blood Pressure

Normal Blood Pressure

Another possible reason why the arteries may be too narrow is a diet low in magnesium. This important mineral is responsible for relaxation. It relaxes the muscles, the heart, the bowels (know what I'm saying? ☐), and it **also relaxes the smooth muscles surrounding the arteries**. In fact, cardiologists in a 2015 article[23] showed a **7.0/3.8 mmHg difference in**

blood pressure between people eating magnesium-rich diets and magnesium-poor diets.

Think it makes sense to raise your magnesium intake if you have high blood pressure? You bet it does.

The foods with the highest magnesium content are **Brazil nuts (get at least 6 nuts), almonds (get at least 20-25 almonds), and dark chocolate** (the darker, the more magnesium it contains. The minimum is 70% cocoa. Go for 30-60 grams, or 1-2 ounces).

As you can see, the vast majority of reasons behind high blood pressure are just about opening up blood vessels. There are multiple ways of doing that.

There is a natural chemical produced in all of our bodies, called "**nitric oxide**." Another natural chemical in foods, called "**nitrates**" helps the body produce its own nitric oxide. What are foods high in nitrates?

- Beets (a cup a day)
- Spinach (a cup a day)
- Celery (6 stalks per day)
- Lettuce (a cup a day)

In a study on hypertension[24], when people consumed a nitrate-rich drink for 4 weeks, their blood pressure was reduced by 7.7/5.2 mmHg. The nitrate-rich drink was standardized to about 250 mg of nitrate. This amount of nitrate is found in about 100 grams of beets, celery, and spinach.

Another common food that has been well-studied in its effects on high blood pressure is flax seeds. In one study[25], hypertensive **people who ate just 30 grams of flax seeds per day lowered their blood pressure by 15/7 mmHg in 6 months**.

When working with clients, I like to keep it simple. I give them this list of foods, and I ask them to just eat one of those with each meal. They have a quota. And now, you have one too □

If you've read about nutrition for high blood pressure in the past, you must have come across the DASH diet (Dietary Approaches to Stop Hypertension), so if the above looks like the DASH diet to you, it's similar.

The Caffeine Controversy

And now, for one of the least popular sections of this book: **caffeine restriction**. I know, you love your morning cuppa Joe, and you need a little boost in the afternoon, when your energy levels are down, but you keep hearing that caffeine increases your blood pressure. Should you cut it out? Or keep it? Let's look at what the evidence has to say.

Several studies[26], have shown that **caffeine does raise blood pressure**. These studies find that the increase is fairly modest in general (only about 4/2 mmHg), but that's in all people – those with high blood pressure, and those without. If you look only at people who already have pre-existing high blood pressure, they seem to be **more responsive to the effects of caffeine** compared to those without high blood pressure, according to a critical reviews[27,28]. So their blood pressure rises higher than those without high blood pressure.

Now yes, according to recent studies[27], **tolerance to caffeine does develop in some people** (meaning that their blood pressure doesn't rise as much after they've been a regular coffee drinker for a while), but not all people.

How does caffeine raise blood pressure? What's the mechanism? Although it's not 100% clear, the main theories are that it **blocks a chemical called "adenosine."** Adenosine causes the relaxation of blood vessels. So if you **block relaxation, you get the opposite – tension**.

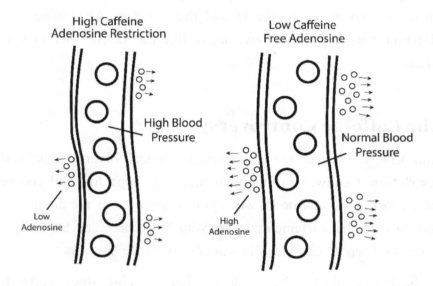

How long does the blood pressure-raising effect of caffeine last? On average, **about 3 hours, but in some people, it's much longer than that**. And remember – those who already have high blood pressure are more sensitive to caffeine than those without high blood pressure.

Want to find out how long caffeine affects *you*, specifically? Here's how you do that:

Step 1: measure your blood pressure.

Step 2: drink your coffee or tea. Drink it in the amounts and concentrations you normally drink.

Step 3: measure your blood pressure every hour, until it returns to normal.

If you want to add validity to this experiment, repeat it on 3-5 different days.

But really, the reason that we're worried about high blood pressure in the first place is because of the risk for heart attacks and strokes. So why not measure whether caffeine actually has an impact on risk of heart attacks and strokes, as opposed to blood pressure? According to one systematic review[29], **although caffeine does raise blood pressure for 3 hours, it does <u>not</u> raise the risk of heart attacks and strokes**. Isn't that great news? Want to go and celebrate with a coffee?

What do we make of all this information? If you don't already have high blood pressure, drinking caffeine won't give you high blood pressure. Enjoy. But if you already have pre-existing high blood pressure, drinking caffeine will raise your blood pressure for a few hours. If you're drinking 2 or more cups a day, your blood pressure may be elevated for all of your waking hours. Also, keep in mind that most studies looking at the effects of caffeine use a dose of 250-300 mg/day. That's about 2 cups of coffee. If you're drinking more than that, there's no great evidence to say if it's still neutral, or starts to become harmful.

Overall, if you want to be super safe, and you think you can handle it, either stop drinking it, or stick to decaf. If you want to go with what the evidence says right now (remember, evidence changes all the time), you can have up to 2 cups of coffee per day relatively safely.

Now, what about tea? I mean, tea has caffeine as well, doesn't it? Yes, it does, but paradoxically, although drinking **tea raises blood pressure in the short term** (by a lot, by the way. About 5/3 mmHg for green tea, and 10/5 mmHg for black tea), for up to 30 minutes (according to an article[30] published on the *"Effects On Blood Pressure Of Drinking Green And Black Tea"*), it seems to return back to baseline by about an hour.

However, the real question is not so much the short-term effects of tea, but the long-term effects. The long-term effects of tea are quite favourable. One systematic review[31] found that consumption of **green tea lowers systolic blood pressure by a modest amount** (about 2 mmHg). Black tea also lowers it by a similar amount, although also appears to have a small effect on diastolic blood pressure as well, according to data gathered[32].

But the **real winner of all teas is hibiscus tea**. In a 2009 study[33] published, when people with pre-hypertension and mild hypertension drank 3 cups per day for 6 weeks, their blood pressure dropped by an average of 7/3 mmHg.

Long Term Effects of Tea

Black Tea	Green Tea	Hibiscus Tea
-2 / 0 mmHg	-2 / 0 mmHg	-7 / -3 mmHg

If you're wondering "what about decaffeinated green of black tea?", the answer is that we have no research investigating their effects on high blood pressure. But I will give my opinion. Tea doesn't lower blood pressure because of its caffeine content. Rather, it lowers blood pressure in spite of it. Tea contains a natural chemical in it called "theanine", which calms down the nervous system. That's one mechanism that we are aware of. However, there are likely other natural chemicals in tea that in combination with each other, lower blood pressure.

Which Foods to Eat Less of

We all know that sodium/salt is a common recommendation for lowering blood pressure. Why? Because **where sodium goes, water goes**. If sodium goes into your arteries, water goes along with it, which increases the volume of fluid inside the arteries. That causes the fluid to push harder.

That's why lowering sodium intake is a common recommendation. Most canned/boxed foods (outside of fruits and veggies) are high in sodium, but on the natural side of things, pickles (actually, anything pickled) and olives are high in sodium.

Not everyone with high blood pressure needs to restrict sodium. In some people, it doesn't have much of an effect, whereas in others it has a very large effect. The way to figure it out is to **try a low-sodium diet for 1 week (that's 1500 mg of sodium per day or less), and see the differences in your blood pressure. If it dropped by at least 5-6 mmHg, it's a good idea to stay on the low sodium diet**.

But if it didn't drop much, you're probably fine to keep it in there.

Some of you may be wondering "are there differences between the different types of salt (Himalayan salt, sea salt, Celtic salt, etc.)?" Unfortunately, there's no research that I'm aware of investigating the effects of these different types of salt on blood pressure. So this is where I give my 2 cents. The ultimate determinant of the blood pressure-raising effect of salt is the sodium content.

One gram of regular table salt (about a fifth of a teaspoon) has about 387 mg of sodium. One gram of sea salt has about 468 mg of sodium. One gram of Himalayan (pink) salt has about 283 mg of sodium. So you're thinking "ah-ha! I'll just switch to Himalayan salt, because it has less sodium." But keep in mind that because it has less sodium, you'll just have to use more of it to get the same taste as table salt.

Very often, people are quick to point out that Himalayan salt has more potassium, magnesium and calcium than regular table salt, and it does. One gram of Himalayan salt has a whopping 4 mg of calcium (we need 1200-1500 mg/day), 0.2 mg of magnesium (we need 300-500 mg/day), and 3.5 mg of potassium (we need up to 4700 mg/day). So for all intents and purposes, the differences between the different kinds of salt is negligible… in my opinion.

But if you really want to be sure, you can do your own study on yourself.

For a week, keep track of how much salt you use (whatever type of salt you do use), and concurrently measure your blood pressure. The following week, use the same amount, but of a different type of salt, and keep measuring your blood pressure. If it dropped, you know that the new type of salt you used has more favourable effects on your blood pressure. If it didn't drop, you know it didn't work.

Alcohol

While with caffeine, I was able to at least give you some good news, with alcohol, I can't do the same. The research is quite clear on alcohol. At best, it's neutral (note: "neutral" does not mean "healthy." Neutral just means it doesn't make your health worse, but it doesn't make it better). At worst, **it raises blood pressure**. And the "at best" scenario is only if you drink no more than 1-2 drinks per day if you're a man, and 1 drink per day if you're a woman.

Beer

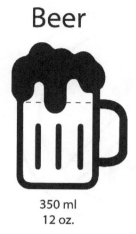

350 ml
12 oz.

Wine

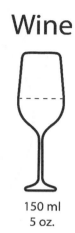

150 ml
5 oz.

Just so we're all on the same page, how much is a "drink"? It's 14 grams of pure alcohol. This amount is found in about 350 ml (12 oz.) of beer and 150 ml (5 oz.) of wine.

Any more than those numbers, and blood pressure starts to rise according to studies[34].

The primary theory on the reasons that alcohol raises blood pressure, according to the study[35] on alcohol induced hypertension, are that it **decreases nitric oxide** – a chemical needed for the blood vessels to dilate. The second reason is that alcohol damages the inside of blood vessels, which also **stiffens them,** and makes them unable to dilate.

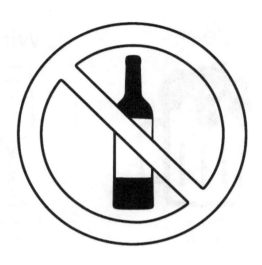

AVOID ALCOHOL

Food Sensitivities

While most of what I write about has substantial research behind it, food sensitivities don't fit in that category. But I feel the need to write about it, since there is good mechanistic evidence.

First – what's a food sensitivity? Is it the same as an allergy? Not quite. **A sensitivity is like a low-grade allergy**. The difference is that allergies are severe and immediate. For instance, you eat a peanut, and within seconds, your throat shuts. Or you eat shellfish, and within a few minutes, your skin breaks out in hives. Those are outright allergies. By contrast, **sensitivities are subtle and delayed**. For instance, you eat gluten (usually found in wheat, rye and barley), and next day, your joints are stiff. Or you drink dairy, and 2 days later, your nose is congested.

Because sensitivities are subtle and delayed, you may go your whole life, and not know you have it. And it's not quite so easy to figure out, since it may be otherwise healthy foods, like spinach and chicken.

Why would food sensitivities raise blood pressure? If you're eating something that you like, but doesn't work so well for your body, it **releases too much cortisol**, which could narrow the arteries. The other mechanism is you could **retain water** from that food, so you have too much fluid inside your arteries.

So investigating what your own food sensitivities are is certainly worth a shot if you have high blood pressure. How would you figure that out?

In order to investigate food sensitivities in my clients, I prefer to use a test that measures IgG, IgA, IgM and IgE which is a laboratory test that accurately pinpoints food sensitivities. This test lists approximately 200 different foods. There are pros and cons to this method. The pros: **speed** (5-7 business days) and **accuracy** (although older IgG-only tests had a lot of inaccurate results, newer tests from advanced laboratories are much better). The cons: **price**. It ain't cheap (typically between $450 and $1800 at the time of this writing).

If you prefer to not do the lab test, then you can go the route of doing an **elimination diet**. The downside of this option, although it may cost a lot less, is that you have to **exercise self-discipline**. To accurately find out what you are sensitive to, you *have to* eliminate the most common allergens for the four-week test period.

This means reading labels and being very careful about what you eat. That leaves you with plenty of vegetables (except for potatoes, tomatoes, bell peppers, egg plants, corn, and chili peppers), most meats (except pork), and most nuts and seeds, in addition to all fruit. You can eat any of these in unlimited quantities. You should not go hungry -this is important.

What do you eliminate? Start with the most common allergens in North America, which are gluten, dairy, sugar, corn, and soy. Also, if you want to make it specific to you, **eliminate/replace the foods that you eat on a regular basis**. Do you have chicken every day? Try replacing it with turkey for this 4-week period. Do you eat tomatoes daily? Try replacing those with an alternative as well. It's often the foods you eat most often (even if they are otherwise healthy foods) that you are likely to be sensitive to.

After removing all of these foods for 4 weeks, on day 29, you **bring back just 1 of them, and note your symptoms**. Note things like joint pain, skin quality, bowel movements, nasal congestion, mood, and most importantly, **measure your blood pressure**. If all of those are unchanged when you bring back a food that you eliminated, you can keep it in. After 3 days, bring back another food that you eliminated. Continue to bring back 1 food every 3 days, until they've all returned.

Now, what do you do if you bring back an eliminated food, and you do see changes in symptoms? Remove it for another month, and bring it back in again. If it produces the same symptoms (and an elevation in blood pressure) the second time around, it's probably a good idea to keep it out permanently.

Sometimes, something as simple as removing a food that you might have been eating your whole life can normalize your blood pressure relatively quickly (even if it's an otherwise healthy food).

Supplements for
High Blood Pressure

S ome people are taking boatloads of supplements, constantly looking for the magic pill. Others are completely skeptical of supplements, thinking they're just a hoax. The truth is really somewhere in the middle. But make no mistake about it – **there are some very potent, proven supplements out there that can help you lower your blood pressure**. Likewise, there are also tons of supplements that are unproven, and by the end of this chapter, you'll know what works, what doesn't, and what we don't know.

Here's what we'll cover in this chapter:

- Two myths about supplements

- Three reasons why I REALLY like supplements

- How to find the right dose

- Effective supplements for lowering your blood pressure

- Ineffective supplements for lowering your blood pressure

- Unproven supplements

- How to combine supplements

But before we get to it, I have to do the obligatory disclaimer: I don't know you. I don't know your health status, what other supplements and medications you are taking, and other pertinent factors. So before you start taking any of the supplements in this chapter, **speak to a pharmacist first**. A lot of people make the mistake of thinking "supplements are natural, therefore they can't do any harm." And boy, are they wrong. If you're taking a blood pressure-lowering medication, and you combine that with a supplement that lowers your blood pressure as well, you might have a combined effect, and your blood pressure would drop too low. If it drops too low, you might faint.

Or, a supplement that you're taking may negate the effects of a medication that you're taking, so your blood pressure wouldn't lower at all.

So again, speak to a pharmacist before you start taking any of these supplements.

With that disclaimer out of the way, let's get to it!

Supplement Myths

Myth #1: Supplements Don't Work

For someone to believe this one, they'd really have to completely ignore the mountains of research done over the decades that supplements do work. That's not to say that every single supplement on the market works. And that's not to say that every supplement works in 100% of people. But to make a blanket statement that there isn't a single supplement out there that works is just plain false.

Then there's the cousin – "**it's just a placebo effect**." First of all, no it's not. In double-blind, placebo-controlled studies, the term "placebo-controlled" means that one group of participants in the study are getting a placebo, and the other is getting the real supplement, and consistently, **the right supplement outperforms the placebo**. Therefore it can't be the placebo effect.

Second of all, even if it was a placebo effect, so what? The placebo effect is a real, measurable effect. If your blood pressure went down, whether due to something real, or something in your mind, who cares about the reason? You're forgetting the main point – **your blood pressure went down!**

Myth #2: You Have to Make Dietary Changes First

False **again**. In most studies, researchers specifically tell participants not to make any dietary changes when they're taking supplements. Why? Because if you start taking a supplement, and you change your diet at the same time, you don't know if the effect was caused by the supplement, by the diet, or both.

And **even in the absence of any dietary changes, some supplements work**. Again, that's not to say that every supplement works (we'll cover what works and what doesn't later in this chapter), but those that do work do so in the absence of any dietary changes.

Three Reasons Why I Really Like Supplements

As you can tell, I'm a big fan of supplements. There are 3 reasons for this. In no particular order:

Reason #1: Effectiveness

As I mentioned in the previous section, the supplements that work do so in their own right, in the absence of any dietary changes. Would you get an additive effect if you combined them with changes in exercise and nutrition? Sure. But you still get anywhere from a moderate to a large effect on your blood pressure without any other changes.

Reason #2: Compliance

If you've ever been on a diet before, you know that dietary changes are hard. If you've been eating a certain way for 40, 50, 60 years or more, it's very hard to change those long-standing habits.

But taking a pill, powder or liquid? That's easy! Most people have near-100% compliance with that. Whereas dietary changes, given that 80-95% of people who lose weight regain it, don't have anywhere near the same compliance level.

Reason #3: Speed

Some supplements work quickly (in a matter of hours), and other supplements take a few weeks of taking them regularly to have any effect. But even if a supplement takes a month to work, that's relatively fast for most people.

How to Find the Right Supplement Dose

With any supplement, you want to make sure you're taking a dose high enough that it's effective, but low enough that it doesn't cause any adverse effects.

There are a couple of factors that go into figuring out the optimal dose for you:

Factor #1: **your own bodyweight**. The more you weigh, the more of a dose you need.

Factor #2: your **personal reactivity** to it. Some people are highly responsive to supplements, and others aren't.

To figure out the right dose for you, here's a step-by-step process you should use:

Step 1: **start at the dose that it says on the label** of whatever supplement you're taking. Stay at that dose for 2 weeks. Note if it had the desirable effect (did it lower your blood pressure?)

Step 2: **raise the dose by the smallest possible increment** for another 2 weeks. Note if after an additional 2 weeks the effect increased, or it stayed the same. If the effect stayed the same, go back to the dose used in step 1. If the effect increased, move on to step 3

Step 3: keep repeating step 2 until either the effect has maxed out (no larger drops in blood pressure despite larger doses), or you've reached the maximal safe dose.

Step 4: after about 1-2 months, try reducing the dose by the smallest possible increment. If the blood pressure is unchanged after 2 weeks at the lower dose, reduce it again by the smallest possible increment. However, if the blood pressure went up after you reduced the dose, raise it back up again.

If you want to add an additional layer of certainty, you can speak to your doctor or naturopathic doctor about running nutrient testing (one of the most standard tests for it is called an "organic acids profile").

Effective Supplements

Now, we get to the fun part: the supplements that work. The supplements listed here have been shown to work by multiple studies, in humans. I emphasize "in humans", because a lot of supplements go to market prematurely. They're shown to work in either mice/rats, or petri dishes. But not people. Each supplement listed in this section has been shown to work in people, across more than 1 study.

Potassium

One large meta-analysis[36] showed a blood pressure reduction of 8.2/4.5 mmHg from supplementing with potassium. Another meta-analysis[37] found similar reductions.

How it works: if you've read the chapter on nutrition, then you already know how it works. If you haven't, here's the mechanism: when you supplement with potassium, it keeps sodium in balance, which in turn prevents excess water from accumulating inside the arteries. Additionally, **potassium opens up blood vessels in its own right**.

Upper limit: 2500 mg/day.

Symptoms of toxicity:

- Heart palpitations
- Nausea
- Vomiting
- Difficulty breathing
- Numbness and tingling

Magnesium

One narrative review[38], showed a blood pressure reduction of about 4/3 mmHg from magnesium supplementation. Though to be fair, the average dose of magnesium used was about 370 mg/day. Higher doses usually show greater reductions.

Types of magnesium that are effective: magnesium glycinate, magnesium orotate, and magnesium taurate.

How it works: magnesium helps the smooth muscle surrounding arteries relax, which increases the space inside an artery.

Upper limit: 350 mg of actual magnesium. The reason I say "actual" magnesium is because when you get 350 mg of magnesium in supplements, it's not all magnesium. The majority of it is the chelate. So when you get 350 mg of magnesium glycinate, the label will break down how much of the dose is actual magnesium, and how much is other "stuff."

Symptoms of toxicity:

- Excessively low blood pressure
- Diarrhea
- Depression
- Lethargy
- Nausea
- Feelings of weakness

Allicin (AKA Aged Garlic Extract)

In an analysis review[39], when people with high blood pressure supplemented with aged garlic extract, their blood pressure dropped by an average of 16.3/9.3. Quite impressive, right?

How it works: if you'll remember from chapter 2, garlic has a number of different mechanisms:

- It's a natural beta blocker – it blocks the receptors for adrenaline, preventing the blood vessels from closing

- It inhibits the hormone angiotensin, which causes the constriction of blood vessels. What you have done is you blocked constriction and you get dilation.

- It prevents the smooth muscle surrounding arteries from contracting

- It contains nitric oxide, which also dilates blood vessels

Upper limit: according to Examine.com[40], garlic extract should not exceed 5% of the diet. So that's 17 grams for a 150-pound person, 22.7 grams for a 200-pound person, and 28.4 grams for a 250-pound person.

Symptoms of toxicity: unknown

Nitrate/Beetroot Juice

In two different meta-analyses (one on the effects of dietary nitrate supplements on blood pressure[41] and another on Inorganic Nitrate and beet root juice on blood pressure[42],), nitrate supplementation lowered blood pressure by about 4/2 mmHg, and there was no difference between using it for 3 days and 3 months.

How it works: supplemental nitrate gets converted into another chemical called "nitric oxide", which causes the smooth muscles surrounding arteries to relax, and that opens up the arteries.

Upper limit: 12.8 mg/kg

Symptoms of toxicity:

- Weakness

- Shortness of breath without much exertion

- Loss of coordination

Olive Leaf Extract

In a study[43], olive leaf extract lowered blood pressure by 11.5/4.8 mmHg, when taken at a dose of 500 mg, twice a day.

How it works: olive leaf extract inhibits the hormone angiotensin, which causes the constriction of blood vessels. So you block constriction and you get dilation.

Upper limit: unknown. Studies have gone up to 1000 mg/day, without noting any symptoms of toxicity

Symptoms of toxicity: unknown, but theorized that it can cause stomach pain and headaches.

Greens Drinks (Fruit and Vegetables Powders)

In a recent research article[44], a greens drink lowered blood pressure by 12.4/7.1 mmHg when taken daily for 90 days. This is without a change/loss in weight.

How it works: because greens drinks are a mix of different vegetables and fruits, they have all the mechanisms of action of the previous supplements:

- They are natural beta blockers – they block the receptors for adrenaline, preventing the blood vessels from closing

- They inhibit the hormone angiotensin, which causes the constriction of blood vessels; So you block constriction and you get dilation.

- They prevent the smooth muscle surrounding arteries from contracting

- They contain nitric oxide, which also dilates blood vessels

Upper limit: unknown

Symptoms of toxicity:

- Diarrhea

- Bloating

- Indigestion

- Fatigue

Fish Oil

One meta synthesis[45] found that when people with high blood pressure supplemented with fish oil at a dose of 3-7 g/day, their blood pressure dropped by 2.9/1.6 mmHg. And when they supplemented with 15 g/day, their blood pressure dropped by 8.1/5.8 mmHg.

Because **fish oil quality varies so much from company to company** (in some stores, fish oil is already rancid by the time it's on the shelf… only you don't know it, because it's covered up by the smell of lemon or orange), I'll tell you what to look for.

- You want an **opaque container**

- You want something that is **stored in refrigerated temperatures** (room temperature or higher speeds up the rancidity of oil)

- For smaller doses (under 5 g/day), capsules will do. For larger doses (over 5 g/day), liquid is better

How it works: according to one study on Omega-3 fatty acids[46], fish oil lowers blood pressure by activating potassium channels (that means that the cells can take in more potassium, which counterbalances sodium).

Upper limit: unknown.

Symptoms of toxicity:

- Oil leakage out of anus

- Bleeding

- Diarrhea

- Insomnia

- Indigestion

- Vomiting

CoEnzyme Q10 (CoQ10)

CoQ10 is an antioxidant and a natural chemical found in cells. Together with other processes and chemicals, it's **responsible for energy production**.

One meta-analysis[47] found that people with high blood pressure who supplemented with CoQ10 lowered their blood pressure by as much as 17/10 mmHg. The full effects take several months to be actualized, and the doses varied from 75-360 mg/day. A study[48] on the effect of coenzyme

Q10 in physical exercise, hypertension and heart failure, found fairly similar results (blood pressure drops around 16/10 mmHg).

How it works: CoQ10 inhibits the hormone angiotensin, which causes the constriction of blood vessels. So you block constriction and you get dilation. Additionally, it stabilizes calcium channels, preventing calcium from binding to the calcium receptors, and causing contraction of the smooth muscles surrounding arteries.

Upper limit: 1200 mg/day

Symptoms of toxicity:

- Loss of appetite
- Heartburn
- Diarrhea
- Nausea

Ineffective Supplements

Now you know all the supplements that are proven to lower blood pressure (at the time of this writing). There are also lots of supplements said to lower blood pressure, but either don't do so by a great extent, or don't do so at all. That doesn't mean they have no benefit for other reasons, but as far as blood pressure is concerned, they are proven ineffective (though that doesn't stop a lot of supplement manufacturers from putting them into blood pressure-lowering formulas, and claiming they work, despite evidence to the contrary).

Grape Seed Extract

Grape seed extract is one of those where we're not really sure whether it's effective or not. One meta-analysis[49], showed a reduction of 1.54 mmHg, which is not terribly effective. But a different meta-analysis[50], showed varying levels of effectiveness (from not effective at all, up to moderately effective), based on dose, how high the blood pressure was to begin with, and how long it was taken for.

How it works: grape seed extract increases nitric oxide in the body, which dilates blood vessels.

Since it's pretty safe, and you'd like to try it on yourself, to see whether it works for you or not, here's what you need to know:

Upper limit: unknown, but to my knowledge, the highest used dose in research was 2000 mg/day.

Symptoms of toxicity:

- Dizziness

- Nausea

- Headache

Arginine

To be honest, arginine is straddling the border between effective and ineffective, but my choice was to put it in this section, for a few reasons:

1. The dose needed for it to lower blood pressure is quite high. Most research sees the best effects at 10-24 grams/day. Most commercially-available arginine supplements come in doses of 500 mg. So you'd have to pop 20-48 pills per day to have a blood pressure-lowering effect.

2. It doesn't do so reliably in most people, even at the right dose.

3. The degree to which it lowers blood pressure isn't huge. For systolic blood pressure, it's 2.2-5.4 mmHg. For diastolic blood pressure, it's 2.7-3.1 mmHg, according to observations[51].

How it works: arginine stimulates the body to produce nitric oxide, which dilates blood vessels.

Upper limit: unknown, but most studies don't go above 20-24 grams/day

Symptoms of toxicity:

- Diarrhea
- Low blood pressure
- Abdominal pain
- Bloating
- Airway inflammation

Citrulline

Citrulline is an amino acid that is a precursor to arginine. But just like arginine's effect is inconsistent and questionable, so is citrulline's. In one meta synthesis[52], citrulline had no effect on blood pressure.

There's no upper limit and toxicity listed for citrulline because it's not effective, so there's no need to take it.

Folic Acid

Folic acid is one of the B vitamins (B9).

In one narrative review[51], high-dose folic acid supplementation lowered blood pressure by only 2.03/0.01 mmHg.

There's no upper limit and toxicity listed for folic acid because it's not effective, so there's no need to take it.

Unproven Supplements

Very often, people confuse "unproven" with "ineffective." But they're not the same. Ineffective means "it doesn't work." But **"unproven" means "we don't know if it works."** Either studies haven't been done, or the studies had methodological flaws that make conclusions about effectiveness very difficult.

Fortunately, you don't care about averages – you care about you. You can do your own "study" on yourself. My first instinct with clients is to recommend what's proven, and has a high degree of efficacy. But if you want to give these a try, go for it (after a conversation with a pharmacist, of course). You will learn about how these supplements affect your body, faster than it takes to conduct a study.

Hawthorn Extract

Hawthorn is a plant in the berry family. The extract takes the "active ingredient", thought to lower blood pressure, and standardizes it to a certain dose.

In one systematic review[53] on the effects of Hawthorn and blood pressure, researchers saw that the majority (so not all of them) of studies (which is only 4) found it beneficial for high blood pressure, but because of the vast differences in people's responses and study design, it was difficult to pin down an average by which blood pressure is reduced.

How it works:

- Hawthorn is an antioxidant

- Hawthorn stimulates nitric oxide production, which opens up blood vessels

- To a small extent, it inhibits the hormone angiotensin

Upper limit: unknown, but the highest dose used in research is 1800 mg/day.

Symptoms of toxicity:

- Nausea

- Headache

- Dizziness

- Fatigue

- Digestive problems

Valerian Root

To my knowledge, there aren't any studies on how valerian root affects blood pressure. It's been studied in areas more to do with things like sleep, PMS, and anxiety. But even there, it hasn't shown serious effectiveness.

How it works: for things like anxiety, sleep and PMS, it works by stimulating the body to release more GABA (gamma amino butyric acid), which is a neurotransmitter (brain chemical) that causes relaxation. How it works for high blood pressure: we don't know.

Upper limit: unknown, but the highest dose used in research has been 900 mg/day.

Symptoms of toxicity:

- Hangover-like feeling

- Headache

- Insomnia

- Sedation

Carnitine

Carnitine is an amino acid, and supplementally, it comes in 2 forms: l-carnitine, and acetyl-l-carnitine (ALCAR). The only difference is that ALCAR crosses the blood-brain barrier (the blood-brain barrier is a collection of cells that separates the substances in the blood that can get through to the brain, and the ones that can't).

Very little research has been done on either one when it comes to high blood pressure (the majority of research on carnitine is in the areas of weight loss, exercise and athletic performance. The short version: it's not terribly effective for any of them), so it's hard to make any conclusions.

The only study[54] which adequately links the variables, that I'm aware of that looked at the effects of ALCAR on high blood pressure showed no effects when taken at a dose of 2000 mg/day for 6 months. In this study, ALCAR was taken together with simvastatin (Zocor), so we don't know if there was an interaction between the two.

As for L-carnitine, one meta-analysis[55], showed it to be ineffective in lowering blood pressure when taken at a dose of 2000 mg/day.

How it works: we know how it's supposed to work for weight loss and exercise tolerance, but it's still not totally clear the mechanisms by which it's supposed to lower blood pressure (if it does so at all).

Upper limit: the highest level I've seen used in research is 100 mg/kg/day.

Symptoms of toxicity:

- Diarrhea

- Vomiting

- Nausea

- Abdominal cramping

How to Combine Supplements

You might have looked through this list of supplements, seen which one appeals to you, and starting taking it. But then, you might have had a thought: "if supplement X decreases blood pressure by ___ mmHg, supplement Y decreases blood pressure by ___ mmHg, and supplement Z decreases blood pressure by ___ mmHg, I'll just take them all at the same time."

Or you might be a "why choose" type of person, and decided to take all of them.

Don't.

Usually these **supplements are studied in isolation, and how your body would react if you were to take two or more at the same time is**

unknown. They might have beneficial effects (that's what you're hoping for). But they might just cancel each other out. Or they might have synergistic effects, and drop your blood pressure too low, which would make you more prone to fainting, weakness, lethargy, etc.

To intelligently combine supplements, follow these steps:

Step 1: pick a supplement that you want to try.

Step 2: follow the steps from the section on *how to find the right supplement dose*

Step 3: once you've found the right dose, stay there for 1-2 weeks, or until your blood pressure stabilizes.

Step 4: add another supplement, and repeat step 2

With each new supplement you add, keep monitoring your blood pressure, to see if that supplement works for you (if it lowers your blood pressure more than the supplement(s) that you're already taking) or if it negates the effects of the previous supplements.

It may be best to work with a medical professional who is knowledgeable when it comes to supplements, for the very important reason that supplements are rarely studied together, so little is known how they interact with each other when more than one is taken at a time.

Sleep

A lot of people are not getting the needed amount of sleep. Not only that, but they puff out their chest, proudly stating "**I can get by on 5 or 6 hours of sleep.**"

Well, that's not exactly true. Just because it's not instantly killing you doesn't mean it's good for you. In fact, it may be a significant contributor to your high blood pressure.

That's what we'll discuss in this chapter:

- How bad sleep affects your blood pressure
- The connection between sleep apnea and high blood pressure
- Healthy behaviors that improve your sleep quality
- Supplements for sleep

How Bad Sleep Affects Your Blood Pressure

The connection between sleep and blood pressure has been studied extensively. In one large study[56], of 1741 subjects, **those who slept between 5 and 6 hours per night had a 250% higher chance of developing high blood pressure compared to those who slept over 6 hours**. Those who slept less than 5 hours had a 410% higher chance of developing high blood pressure.

Another very large study[57] on sleep duration and hypertension, of over 700,000 people also found a strong relationship between sleep duration and high blood pressure: **the less you sleep, the higher the chance of high blood pressure**.

In fact, in one very interesting study aimed at sleep and its effect on blood pressure[58], participants had extended their time in bed by 1 hour. Of that hour, 35 minutes were spent asleep. In 6 weeks, they lowered their blood pressure by 14/8 mmHg (oh, and they also lost 1.3% body fat in that time. Nice bonus).

Anyways, suffice it to say that sleep is very important to your health. It's not just a passive rest. **Your body and brain are hard at work normalizing body functions while you're sleeping**.

Mechanisms

We know that getting too little sleep is not good for your blood pressure, but why? There are 3 different reasons:

1. Getting low amounts of sleep is considered to be a physically stressful condition. **When you're under physical stress, you crave more salt**, according to a study[59] on mental stress on various living things, ranging from mice to humans. You either go for salty snacks, or you salt your food more than when you're not under stress. We know that salt increases water retention, which raises blood pressure.

2. Another study[60] exploring the causes of hypertension, found that getting **inadequate sleep causes thickening of one of the heart walls** (left ventricular hypertrophy). If the heart gets thicker and more "muscular", it pushes blood harder. If it pushes blood harder, arteries also have to adapt by thickening as well.

Normal Heart
Normal Blood Pressure Output

More Muscular Heart
Stronger Blood Pressure Output

Normal Thickness Arteries

Thicker Arteries

Normal Blood Pressure

High Blood Pressure

3. One more study[61] found that **inadequate sleep increases insulin levels**. High insulin levels cause hardening of the arteries (that process is called "atherosclerosis"). Harder arteries require more pressure to get blood through them.

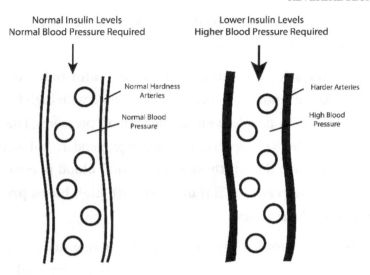

4.   To piggyback on the previous point, inadequate sleep can causes insulin resistance, according to one study[62] . Insulin resistance is when your body doesn't "hear" the message of insulin (insulin tells cells to "open their doors", and let sugar out of the blood, and inside the cells). There are a number of ways by which insulin resistance leads to hypertension. You hold on to more sodium, you grow the smooth muscles surrounding the arteries (you don't want to grow these muscles), and you have higher levels of cortisol and adrenaline.

The Connection Between Sleep Apnea and High Blood Pressure

Now that I've (hopefully) convinced you of the importance of sleep, what should you do? If you go to sleep late voluntarily, stop it. Listen to your mom from when you were a teenager: go to bed on time. Go to bed at the same time every night.

But if you don't sleep well, and it's not by choice, it's worthwhile **getting tested for sleep apnea**.

Sleep apnea is a huge underlying contributor to hypertension, and it's not looked at enough. In one study[63], people with high blood pressure were compared to people without high blood pressure. The researchers made sure that both groups had the same age, gender, and weight. But the big difference was this: **of those with normal blood pressure, only 4% of them had sleep apnea. But of those with high blood pressure, 38% of them had sleep apnea**.

This was in "normal" hypertension. But in one study of what's called "resistant hypertension", the difference is even more stark. First of all, what's "resistant hypertension?" **Resistant hypertension is defined as having blood pressure over 140/90, despite taking at least 3 medications for high blood pressure, at their maximal doses**. In short: resistant hypertension is when medications aren't lowering blood pressure. In people with this type of hypertension, as much as 83% of them have sleep apnea, according to a study[64] on unrecognized sleep apnea.

So the first step would be to go to your doctor, and ask for the test (it's called a "sleep study"). This is even if:

- You don't snore

- You're not sleepy during the day

- You don't wake up with a dry mouth

The typical treatment for sleep apnea is the use of a CPAP machine (continuous positive airway pressure). It allows you to sleep at night much more restfully. In a study[65] on untreated hypertension and difficulty in breathing, **when people with high blood pressure used a CPAP**

machine for 3 weeks, their blood pressure dropped by an average of 7.8/5.3 mmHg.

This is a worthwhile condition to treat, because its effects are so far-reaching. Sleep apnea is either a contributing factor or a root cause for:

- High blood pressure
- Stroke
- Heart attacks
- Heart failure
- Depression
- Migraines
- Diabetes

  …and more.

So the message is simple: get tested. If you have sleep apnea, get treated.

The Basics of Sleep Hygiene

Now, what if you've been tested, and you don't have sleep apnea? Are you off the hook? Not so fast. If you don't take your sleep seriously, you should. Just think about it: if you're supposed to spend about one third of your life asleep, that must mean that it's pretty important. So treat it with the care that it deserves.

Here are the bare basics that you need to do to optimize your sleep:

1. **Bedtime regularity**. Go to bed at the same time each day, including weekends. When you go to bed at different times, it

messes up your circadian rhythms. Imagine going to bed at 10:30PM one day, and 12:30AM the next day. To your body, it's the equivalent of going to bed in different time zones.

2. **Blue light**. In the entire spectrum of light, blue light is meant to wake you up. Great when it's time to wake up, but not so good when it's time to go to sleep. A study on blue light and Insomnia[66], has shown that when blue light is blocked in the hours before bed, people fall asleep faster, and sleep longer. There are a couple of ways to block blue light:

a. Wear blue-light blocking glasses (check them out on Amazon) about an hour before bed.

b. Modern smart phones and computers have blue light settings built in, so just figure out how to change the blue light settings on your phone and computer.

3. To piggyback on the previous point, you want **complete darkness**. As dark as possible. You shouldn't see moonlight, streetlights, or anything else. The more light there is in the room, the less melatonin you make (the hormone you release during sleep).

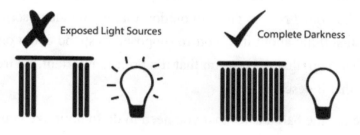

4. **Temperature**. Your room should be cool. Maybe 1-2 degrees Celsius (about 2-4 degrees Fahrenheit) lower than your daytime temperature.

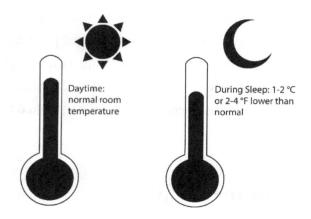

5. **Caffeine**. If you can drink it, and fall asleep just fine, do whatever you want. But if you drink it and it keeps you awake, keep it far enough from bedtime.

6. **Don't keep your cell phone in the bedroom** with you. If you use it as an alarm clock, just get an old-school alarm clock.

7. Have your last meal 3-5 hours before bed. The larger the meal, the farther from bedtime it should be, because large meals increase the time it takes to fall asleep.

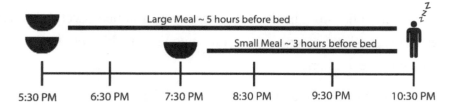

8. **Use your bedroom only for sleep and sex**. If you do your work from your bedroom, it starts to become associated with a time

of focus, not relaxation. Everything that's not sleep and sex should be done in other rooms. Well… you can have sex in other rooms, too.

If you're wondering "can you get too much sleep?", the answer is "yes", although not enough sleep is a far bigger problem, so much more research is devoted to that. Generally speaking, risk of high blood pressure does rise over about 8-9 hours. So if that's you, that should also be looked into. Very often, excessive sleep (hypersomnia) is linked to depression and hypothyroidism.

Supplements for Sleep

If you've implemented all of the suggestions from earlier in this chapter, it should help about 60-80% of you sleep better. But what about the remaining 20-40%? Don't worry, I won't leave you hanging. In this section, I'll show you some supplements to help you sleep.

Magnesium

You might be thinking "but Igor, I already use magnesium, and I'm still having a hard time sleeping." Well, my friend, there may be 2 issues at hand: form and dosage.

If you'll walk into a health food store, you'll notice several different types of magnesium: magnesium oxide, magnesium chloride, magnesium citrate, and a few others.

Different forms of magnesium work on different tissues… and some don't work all that well at all. Like magnesium oxide doesn't get absorbed very well.

Sleep agents

Magnesium glycinate

...ve system. Magnesium taurate ...**magnesium glycinate** affects ...it's the most effective form to

...nents for magnesium. If you're ...vegetables, and don't exercise ...ental magnesium are pretty low ...u're under a lot of stress, and exercise pretty hard, your requirements for magnesium rise (oh, and if you have high blood pressure, your requirements for magnesium are probably higher than for someone without high blood pressure).

So I recommend starting at 300 mg per day, taken after 4 PM in divided doses. If you end up sleeping well at that dose, stick with it. If you still don't sleep well after about a week, increase the dose to 400 mg per day, after 4 PM in divided doses. Keep going up like that until you've either started to sleep well, or you've reached the maximal dose (see the supplement chapter for what the maximal dose is... it's a bit more complex than an actual number).

How Does it Work?

Magnesium works because **it relaxes different tissues of the body**. In this case, we're trying to relax the muscles and nervous system.

Magnesium and calcium are opposite minerals. Calcium helps with contraction and tension. Magnesium helps with relaxation. When there is an imbalance between calcium and magnesium in favour of calcium, you start having a hard time sleeping. But when the two are in balance, you're in good health.

5-HTP

5-HTP is my second most frequently-recommended supplement. I start my clients off at 300-500 mg, and use the same process as with magnesium to figure out the correct dosage.

The way it works is by being a precursor to melatonin, the hormone you release when you're asleep.

5-HTP gets converted to serotonin (AKA "the happy chemical"), which eventually gets converted to melatonin. Therefore it's giving you the raw material necessary to make melatonin.

Melatonin

Lastly, the most common sleep supplement, melatonin. Why is it listed last here? Because it's pretty misunderstood. At my seminars, a lot of people complain to me "I take/took melatonin, but it's not helping me sleep."

Again, there are a couple issues at hand: **form and dosage**.

As a general rule, good supplements *do not* come from drug stores, grocery stores and supermarkets. So if you bought your melatonin there, it explains why it's not working for you.

The **best melatonin is the kind you drop under the tongue**.

In terms of dosage, I start my clients at 500 micrograms, and work them up either to 5 mg, or a dose that works, whichever comes first.

Furthermore, you have to use the right tool for the job. Melatonin's primary function is in helping you fall asleep. It seems to be less effective in helping you stay asleep.

There you have it: our 3 most powerful supplements that we use to help people fall asleep.

You might be asking yourself though "do I need all 3?" The answer is that no single strategy works for 100% of the people, 100% of the time. For the cases when one supplement doesn't work, use a different one.

And again, I want to reiterate what I mentioned at the beginning: supplementation is my second choice in helping people fall and stay asleep.

My first choice is improving sleep hygiene.

Individualization

Y ou've heard the saying "everyone's an individual", but for the most part, it's been just a cliché, with no actionable information.

In this chapter, you'll learn how to tailor the advice in the previous chapters to your body.

As I'm fond of saying in my seminars, "**if you're not assessing, you are guessing**." So start assessing.

What do you assess? Your blood pressure. Measure it twice per day for a week, and track it in an Excel document, or wherever else you want. During this week, don't change anything. Don't change your exercise, nutrition, supplements or medications.

After you've recorded your blood pressure for a week, note a few important measurements:

- Your average blood pressure
- Your highest systolic blood pressure
- Your highest diastolic blood pressure
- Your lowest systolic blood pressure
- Your lowest diastolic blood pressure

Why are we so anal about it, as to separate the systolic and diastolic? Because different approaches may affect one, but not the other.

After that one week of getting a baseline, you can decide what you want to do:

- The scientific approach

- The fast approach

- The hybrid approach

The Scientific Approach

With the scientific approach, you **only make one change at a time**. Pick whatever you want, from any of the previous chapters – pick a supplement, pick a food, pick a form of exercise. Doesn't matter. As long as it's just one.

Implement that consistently for a week, while continuing to track your blood pressure.

If after a week, your blood pressure dropped, keep it going for another week, and another and another, until your blood pressure stabilizes. Once it stabilizes, add to it. Either do more of what you were already doing (so if you were already doing cardio 3 times per week for 30 minutes, try 4 times per week for 30 minutes. Or try 3 times per week for 40 minutes), or keep what you were already doing, and add something different (keep the cardio, and add garlic, for instance).

Once you've done that, keep tracking your blood pressure. **As long as your blood pressure continues to drop, keep what you were doing**. Once your blood pressure has been stable for a week, implement the third change.

Keep going like this until your blood pressure has normalized.

There are advantages and disadvantages to this method.

Advantages:

    1. **Sustainability**: if you implement changes one-by-one, you're more likely to stick with them long term.

    2. **Certainty**: because you're only changing one thing at a time, you know for sure what's driving your results.

    3. **Caution**: your blood pressure is unlikely to drop too much, too fast

Disadvantages:

The only big disadvantage is **speed**. Because you're only making one change at a time, and waiting for results to stabilize, it can take several months to normalize your blood pressure.

The Fast Approach

With the fast approach, **you throw everything in this book at your hypertension at the same time**: exercise, nutrition and supplements.

As you're doing that, keep monitoring your blood pressure twice per day.

But a word of caution: **don't include every single supplement in the supplement chapter here**. You can combine exercise with nutrition, and one supplement, but I wouldn't go above that, because there's the risk of your blood pressure dropping too much, too fast, which can predispose you to fainting, lethargy and weakness.

If your blood pressure normalized after 1-2 weeks, congrats! You're done making changes. If your blood pressure dropped, but hasn't normalized, and is still dropping, don't change anything. Wait for your blood pressure to stabilize before making additional changes. If it's still dropping, and you implement additional changes, it could drop too low.

But if your blood pressure has stabilized after throwing everything at it, and it hasn't normalized yet, try additional measures, like:

- Increasing your exercise

- Increasing the amount of blood pressure-lowering foods you're eating

- Increasing the dose of the supplement that you're currently taking

- Maintaining the same dose of the supplement that you're already taking, and adding another one.

Like the scientific approach, the fast approach does have advantages and disadvantages.

Advantages:

1. The most obvious: it's **fast**. You could literally normalize your blood pressure in 1 week to 1 month.

2. **Motivation**: it's pretty motivating to see fast changes.

Disadvantages:

1. **Speed** can be an advantage, but it can also be a disadvantage. Your blood pressure might drop too quickly, and can predispose you to fainting, lethargy and weakness.

2. **Lack of certainty**: you don't know where the results are coming from. Exercise? Nutrition? Supplements?

3. **Sustainability**: the more changes you make, the less likely you are to stick with them. But about 5% of people have the personality type to make rapid changes and keep them long-term.

The Hybrid Approach

If you want more speed than the scientific approach, but not so fast that it would drop your blood pressure too low, too quickly, the hybrid approach may be for you.

You don't implement changes one by one, as in the scientific approach, but you don't throw everything at it either, as in the fast approach.

You start with just two changes. Pick any two:

- Exercise and nutrition

- Nutrition and 1 supplement

- Exercise and 1 supplement

The rest of the process is the same. After selecting which two changes you'll be making, keep measuring your blood pressure.

As long as it's dropping, don't change anything. It will stop dropping at one of two points:

- Your blood pressure is now normal (around 115/75 mmHg)

- Your blood pressure is lower than before, but still higher than it should be.

If your blood pressure is now normal, you're done. No other changes need to be made for your blood pressure. Of course, if you'd like to make additional changes for reasons other than blood pressure, you're welcome to.

If your blood pressure is still higher than it should be, implement one more new change, and see if that change results in lower blood pressure after a week. If yes, keep it going, until it stabilizes. If not, replace the change you made with a different one.

Approach	Scientific	Fast	Hybrid
Advantages	Sustainable Certain Cautious	Fast Motivating	Balanced in speed, certainty, and motivation
Disadvantages	Slow	Too fast? Uncertain Unsustainable	

How George Lowered His Blood Pressure By 19/15 mmHg in 12 Weeks

M eet George. He's a 47-year-old sales associate at a health food store. He started working with me because he had high blood pressure. Really high. His **average blood pressure was 154/103** when he started working with me. And it's been that way since about 2006-2007.

At the end of 12 weeks, we were able to **drop his blood pressure to an average of 135/88**.

And along with all that, there was a dramatic change in his lifestyle:

- He has more energy

- His outlook is better

- He can handle stress better

- His doctor is no longer on him to get on his medications.

So in this article, I'll talk about:

- How the high blood pressure was affecting George

- What we found during our assessment of George

- What he has tried in the past to bring down his blood pressure

- A week-by-week breakdown of the exact exercise, nutrition and supplementation strategies we used to drop his blood pressure

- A "post-mortem" on what we could have done to get even better results

How the High Blood Pressure Was Affecting George

Even when everything was going fine in George's life, the **blood pressure was causing a lot of stress and anxiety**. He always felt "edgy." Small things would "set him off."

And overall, his **enjoyment of life was limited**, compared to before he had high blood pressure. It was very difficult to wind down after a long day of work, and George's sleep was affected as well (he wasn't sleeping very well).

And you can imagine, being anxious all the time took a lot of energy out of him. So the vicious cycle continued. He was feeling anxious, which is obviously stressful, which raised his blood pressure. But also, the blood pressure was high, which made him anxious.

What George Has Tried in the Past to Lower His Blood Pressure

Of course, with a blood pressure that high, his doctor completely freaked out, and wanted to put him on medications immediately (this was many years ago). George resisted doctor's orders for about 9 years, until he decided to try the medications. They knocked his energy levels right out. They were already low to begin with, and the medication made them even lower.

So he decided to take himself off his medications. The doctor instead put him on water pills, which were much better tolerated.

George has also been a more or less regular exerciser for 30 years, and despite that, his blood pressure was high (mind you, he wasn't doing exercise targeted at lowering blood pressure, the way I describe in chapter 2).

He's also tried dietary changes, and obviously, a lot of supplements.

Despite all those changes, his blood pressure was crazy high (as noted earlier, on average, 154/103).

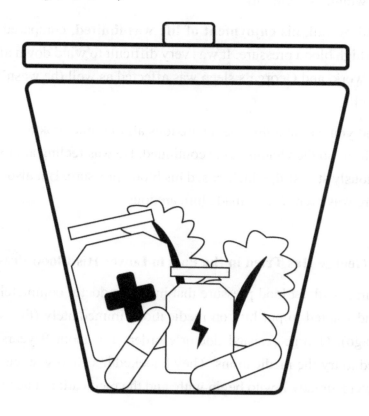

The Assessment

As with all of our clients, we start with measurements. I had George fill out my thorough, 321-symptom questionnaire, and we also did a

biosignature analysis on him. In laymen's terms, biosignature analysis is an assessment we do on our clients that correlates the **location** of someone's body fat to their hormonal profile.

These were our initial findings:

- Out of 16 sections, his highest score was the **blood sugar** section (he scored 21/39. Ideal is 0/39), followed by **essential fatty acids** (the score was 10/22. Again, ideal is 0/22), and then, **adrenals** (score was 31/78). To us, this meant that his high blood pressure was driven by a poor diet, as well as high stress levels.

- There was pain in the left knee

- There was lower back pain when leaning forward

- He was taking A LOT of supplements. Working in a health food store, you get everything at a discount, plus tons of free samples. How can you resist? He was taking CoQ10, a multi-vitamin, a B complex, fish oil, Cardio Mag, turmeric, cocoa powder, testoboost, probiotics, enzymes, sleeping pills and magnesium citrate.

- 3 highest areas in body fat: belly (21 mm), love handle (15 mm), and ribs (15 mm as well)

- Waist circumference: 97 cm (38.2 inches)

In addition to these findings, George was to **measure his blood pressure first thing in the morning, last thing before bed, before exercise, and immediately after exercise.**

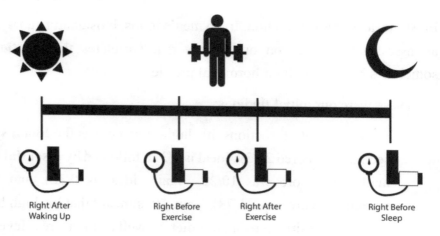

Right After Waking Up   Right Before Exercise   Right After Exercise   Right Before Sleep

Each week, George would keep this information in an Excel file, and at the end of the week, he would send it to me for analysis. This goes back to what I constantly talk about – the importance of measurements.

A Week-By-Week Breakdown of the Strategies We Used to Drop George's Blood Pressure

Before We Started

There was a 3-week gap between when we did George's initial assessment, and when we actually started his program. We were just waiting for George to see his doctor, to give him an update of what he plans to do.

We didn't start until we had the doctor's "all clear."

During this time, I simply had George make one tiny little change:

In addition to his regular exercise routine, he just had to do **6 sets of isometric/static squats, to failure (meaning, until he could no longer hold them), with 2 minutes rest in between sets, 3 times per week**. George's sets lasted between 20 and 40 seconds.

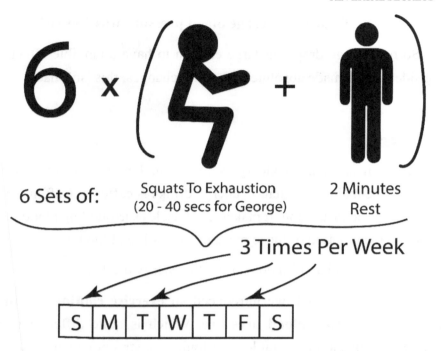

I instructed him not to make any other changes during this time. No changes in nutrition, no changes in supplements.

In the week leading up to our first session, these were the findings:

- George's highest systolic blood pressure was 158, and it only happened once, out of 14 measurements (7 mornings, and 7 evenings).

- George's highest diastolic blood pressure was 104, and it only happened 3 times, out of 14 measurements. All the other measurements were below 104.

- George's lowest systolic blood pressure was 145

- George's lowest diastolic blood pressure was 96

- **George's average blood pressure was 150/101**

So not a huge drop, but large enough to have a tangible effect. And considering we made absolutely no other changes, this isn't bad.

Weeks 1-4

After an analysis of George's food log, I noticed a lot of **energy drinks**. The main ingredient in energy drinks is caffeine. Caffeine has an effect of vasoconstriction. It makes the muscles surrounding blood vessels contract. Contraction of those muscles causes high blood pressure.

Guess what I had him do: cut out the energy drinks.

In addition to that, we introduced an **exercise routine specifically aimed at lowering blood pressure**. Which is quite different than an exercise routine aimed at fat loss, or toning, or strengthening, or anything else. Just as a doctor wouldn't give the same medication for different conditions, **we don't use the same exercise program for different goals**.

I elaborate on the specifics of exercise for high blood pressure, in chapter 2.

What were the results of this?

- The highest systolic blood pressure over this 1-week period was 154, and it only happened once out of 14 measurements (7 mornings, 7 evenings).

- The highest diastolic blood pressure was 104, and it only happened twice out of 14 measurements.

- The lowest systolic blood pressure was 120, and it happened once

- The lowest diastolic blood pressure was 90, and it happened once

- **The average blood pressure over this 1-week period was 147/98**

We stuck with this strategy for the next 4 weeks, because his blood pressure was dropping steadily, so there was no reason to change anything.

Here are his results after week 4:

- The highest systolic blood pressure over this 1-week period was 152, and it only happened once out of 14 measurements (7 mornings, 7 evenings).

- The highest diastolic blood pressure was 101, and it only happened three times out of 14 measurements.

- The lowest systolic blood pressure was 140, and it happened three times

- The lowest diastolic blood pressure was 83, and it happened once

- **The average blood pressure over this 1-week period was 144/95**

But this is pretty similar to his blood pressure from week 3. Which means that he has now been "stuck" at this level for 2 weeks. And his blood pressure was still too high. It was now time to make additional changes.

Weeks 5-6

Now, this is where I instructed George to eat more **potassium-rich foods**.

While sodium restriction is a tried-tested-and-true strategy, according to additional evidence[67], potassium augmentation has a more pronounced effect on blood pressure.

So **why didn't I instruct George to both increase potassium, and decrease sodium? Why just the increase in potassium?** Because by simply adding in more potassium-rich foods, sodium-rich foods automatically decrease. However, the psychological effect of adding something in is much easier than removing something. If I told you not to eat something, you'd want to eat it. But if I gave you a quota of how much to eat of good foods, that "pushes" the "bad stuff" out of your diet.

So now, what did I ask George to eat? I'm sure you're thinking "bananas." I'm not sure why bananas are the poster-child for potassium. Foods like parsley, sun-dried tomatoes, garlic, potatoes, and others are much higher in potassium than bananas. For instance, 100 grams of a banana has about 358 mg of potassium. By comparison, 100 grams of a potato has 421 mg of potassium. And sun-dried tomatoes? In 100 grams, there are 1565 mg. Take that, bananas!

I gave George a quota: **he had to eat 3 potassium-rich foods per day, at least**. If he wanted more, he could have more.

What I secretly wanted was to get his potassium intake up to 4700 mg per day. That's the recommended amount by the American Heart Association. That amount, however, is very difficult to get through food alone. So, I recommended George take **a potassium supplement**.

The results:

- The highest systolic blood pressure was 150, and it only happened once

- The highest diastolic blood pressure was 104, and it only happened once

- The lowest systolic blood pressure was 135

- The lowest diastolic blood pressure was 82

- **The average blood pressure was 142/92**

Weeks 7-8

At this point, I instructed George to add another small exercise to his routine: he was to hold a hand-grip dynamometer, with about 30% of his strength, for 4 sets of 2 minutes, with 2 minutes of rest between sets, 3 times per week.

Again, the rationale behind this kind of exercise is covered in chapter 2.

The results:

- George's highest systolic blood pressure was 146, and it only happened once.

- George's highest diastolic blood pressure was 97, and that only happened once

- George's lowest systolic blood pressure was 132

- George's lowest diastolic blood pressure was 83

- **George's average blood pressure was 141/89**

Week 9-10

By now, we're sitting right around the border of stage 1 hypertension. The official mark of high blood pressure is either a systolic blood pressure of 140, or a diastolic blood pressure of 90. We were now very close to going from "hypertension" to "pre-hypertension."

This week, we added magnesium glycinate. We started with 500 mg, and continued to raise it by 250-500 mg every 2 days, while monitoring for symptoms of toxicity. We saw absolutely no changes in George's blood pressure, until we reached 2000 mg. That's a pretty high dose, indicating a significant magnesium deficiency.

Why did we choose to focus on magnesium in this week? How does magnesium affect blood pressure? **Magnesium is a mineral that relaxes muscles**. So if we would be able to relax the muscles surrounding blood vessels, his blood pressure would drop. In medical terms, magnesium is both a natural **"calcium channel blocker"** (it blocks calcium receptors on the muscles surrounding arteries, which cause contraction), as well as a **"beta blocker"** (it blocks certain receptors for adrenaline), and a **vasodilator** (it opens up blood vessels).

Sure enough, it worked.

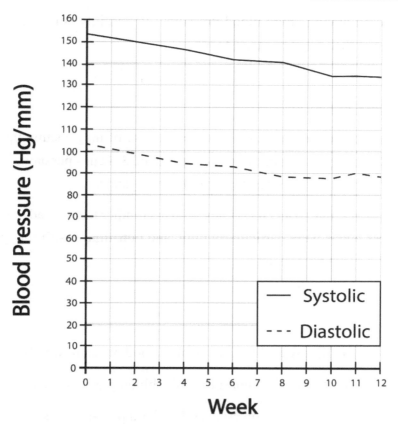

The results:

- George's highest systolic blood pressure was 146

- George's highest diastolic blood pressure was 91

- George's lowest systolic blood pressure was 127

- George's lowest systolic blood pressure was 81

- **George's average blood pressure was 135/87**

And this marks **the first week in 10 years that George was officially no longer "hypertensive."** He no longer met the diagnostic criteria to be

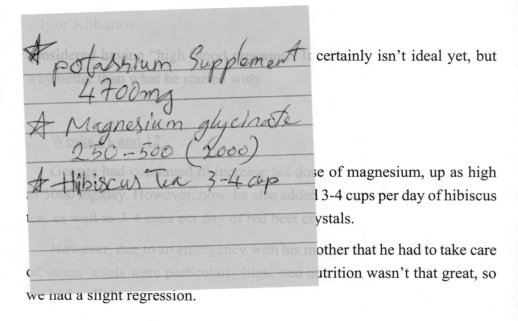

considered buying "high blood pressure" ... certainly isn't ideal yet, but way better than what he started with.

George had continued to increase his dose of magnesium, up as high as 1000 mg/day. However, now he also added 3-4 cups per day of hibiscus tea, as well as 3-4 cups per day of red beet crystals.

However, due to an emergency with his mother that he had to take care of, stress levels were particularly high, and nutrition wasn't that great, so we had a slight regression.

The results:

- George's highest systolic blood pressure was 145
- George's highest diastolic blood pressure was 97
- George's lowest systolic blood pressure was 128
- George's lowest diastolic blood pressure was 84
- **George's average blood pressure was 136/90**

On the surface, it looks like a regression, but we have to take into account the added element of the extra stress with his mother. Ordinarily, under a stressful situation, George's blood pressure would rise a lot more than it did. The fact that his blood pressure didn't rise that high under this situation is a small victory. It means that **even though the stress was there, it was less damaging on his body than if he hadn't been supplementing, and exercising**.

Yes, there's more work to do, to get his blood pressure even better, but not a bad drop in 12 weeks.

Week	Blood Pressure	Changes/Events
Before Training	154/103	none
3 Weeks Before Training	150/101	Introduction of Isometric Squat Exercises
1 - 4	147/98	Reduced Energy Drink Intake, Introduction of Exercise Routine Aimed at Reducing Blood Pressure
End of Week 4	144/95	None
5 - 6	142/92	Increased Potassium-Rich Foods
7 - 8	141/89	Introduction of Dynamometer Exercises
9 - 10	135/87	Introduction of Magnesium Glycinate
11 - 12	136/90	Introduction of Tea, Introduction of Red Beet Crystals, Increased Magnesium Dosage, Added Stress Due to External Factors
End of Week 12	135/88	n/a

What Could Have Gone Better

Point #1: Magnesium

In retrospect, I would have **introduced magnesium supplementation earlier** in the process. The other thing that I would have done differently is be a bit **more aggressive with the dosages**. Once we got to 1000 mg/day, I started getting nervous, even though George was feeling just fine. At that point, I was about to conclude that the magnesium isn't working for George, and was about to drop it altogether.

George suggested trying higher dosages at his own risk. I told him that was his choice, and to just monitor for symptoms of toxicity (like diarrhea, low heart rate, mental sluggishness, etc.). In fact, George didn't experience a blood pressure-lowering effect until he got to 2000 mg. And that was the largest effect of any other strategy that we used. If I had "wimped out" at 1000 mg, George would have missed out on some potent blood pressure lowering effects.

Point #2: Food Sensitivities

Around week 4, I suggested to George to get tested for food sensitivities (which is not the same as allergies). I thought that might have a strong effect on his blood pressure, because if he's constantly eating foods that may be healthy, but he's sensitive to, it could be raising his cortisol, which could in turn raise his blood pressure.

Unfortunately it took 7 weeks to get the results of his test, which was way too long. If I was to do it again, I would have done this earlier in the process.

Point #3: Compliance

George's compliance to my nutrition and exercise recommendations was about 70%. As a result, he missed about 30% of the workouts, and ate/drank things he wasn't supposed to 30% more time than he should have.

It comes as no surprise that better compliance would get better results.

Point #4: Massage, Acupuncture and Meditation

This is more a point of curiosity, whether any of those would have a measurable blood pressure-lowering effect. We did not experiment with those during out 12 weeks together.

So there you have it. The exact week-by-week breakdown of how we turned around George's high blood pressure. All these numbers and analysis are nice, but how does it translate to his quality of life?

- He now has more energy

- He's able to relax and unwind better after a long day at work

- He can sleep better

- He is nicer and kinder to the people around him

- He can provide better care for his mother

If you'd like to get the same, or better results for yourself, you can see if you qualify to work with us (either in person or online) by **sending me an email at Igor@TorontoFitnessOnline.com**

Conclusion

You made it! You finished this book. Or maybe you just flipped to this chapter, because you don't want the science. You just want the bottom line – "what do I do to lower my blood pressure?"

That's what you'll get in this section.

Exercise

- Easy, short, not very time consuming:

    o Squeeze your fists with about 30% force for 2 minutes

    o Relax for 3 minutes

    o Repeat that 3 more times, for a total of 4 sets

    o Do this 3 times per week

- Longer program:

    o Do cardio 3-5 days per week:

        ▪ The intensity should be over 75% of your maximal heart rate (which, theoretically is 220 minus your age. If you're 60, your maximum is theoretically 160, and 75% of that is 120 beats per minute).

        ▪ Do it for about 30-50 minutes

        ▪ The type doesn't matter, whether you're jogging, or cycling, or swimming, or on the elliptical.

    o Do strength training 2-3 times per week:

- Lift weights heavy enough that you can't do them more than 20 times, but light enough that you can do more than 5 times.

- Do 2-5 sets per exercise

- Do 8-10 exercises per workout

Nutrition

- Eat at least 1 of these foods with each meal:
  - Celery
  - Garlic
  - Beets
  - Spinach
  - Sardines
  - Salmon
  - Beef
  - Cheddar cheese
  - Yogurt
  - Dates
  - Prune
  - Potatoes
  - Sun-dried tomatoes
  - Watermelon
  - Parsley

- o Asparagus

Supplements

Supplements That Work:

- Potassium

  - o Don't exceed: 2500 mg/day

- Magnesium glycinate

  - o Don't exceed: 350 mg/day of actual magnesium

- Allicin (AKA aged garlic extract)

  - o Don't exceed:

    - 17 grams if you're 150 pounds

    - 22.7 grams if you're 200 pounds

    - 28.4 grams if you're 250 pounds

- Nitrate/beetroot juice

  - o Don't exceed: 12.8 mg/kg

- Olive leaf extract

  - o Don't exceed: 1000 mg/day

- Greens drinks

- Fish oil

- CoEnzyme Q10 (CoQ10)

  - o Don't exceed: 1200 mg/day

Supplements That Don't Work:

- Grape seed extract

- Arginine

- Citrulline

- Folic acid

Unproven Supplements

- Hawthorn extract

    o Don't exceed: 1800 mg/day

- Valerian root

    o Don't exceed: 900 mg/day

- Carnitine (both L-carnitine, and acetyl-l-carnitine)

    o Don't exceed: 100 mg/kg/day

If you've implemented these changes, and lowered or normalized your blood pressure, I'd love to hear from you. Email me at Igor@TorontoFitnessOnline.com with your results.

Bibilography

1. Brandão Rondon, M. U., Alves, M. J., Braga, A. M., Teixeira, O. T., Barretto, A. C., Krieger, E. M., & Negrão, C. E. (2002). Postexercise blood pressure reduction in elderly hypertensive patients. Journal of the American College of Cardiology, 39(4), 676–682. https://doi.org/10.1016/s0735-1097(01)01789-2

2. Ciolac, E. G., Guimarães, G. V., D Avila, V. M., Bortolotto, L. A., Doria, E. L., & Bocchi, E. A. (2009). Acute effects of continuous and interval aerobic exercise on 24-h ambulatory blood pressure in long-term treated hypertensive patients. International journal of cardiology, 133(3), 381–387. https://doi.org/10.1016/j.ijcard.2008.02.005

3. Eicher, J. D., Maresh, C. M., Tsongalis, G. J., Thompson, P. D., & Pescatello, L. S. (2010). The additive blood pressure lowering effects of exercise intensity on post-exercise hypotension. American heart journal, 160(3), 513–520. https://doi.org/10.1016/j.ahj.2010.06.005

4. Thompson, P. D., Crouse, S. F., Goodpaster, B., Kelley, D., Moyna, N., & Pescatello, L. (2001). The acute versus the chronic response to exercise. Medicine and science in sports and exercise, 33(6 Suppl), S438–S453. https://doi.org/10.1097/00005768-200106001-00012

5. Guidry, M. A., Blanchard, B. E., Thompson, P. D., Maresh, C. M., Seip, R. L., Taylor, A. L., & Pescatello, L. S. (2006). The influence of short and long duration on the blood pressure response to an acute bout of dynamic exercise. American heart journal, 151(6),. https://doi.org/10.1016/j.ahj.2006.03.010

6. Zeppilli, P., Vannicelli, R., Santini, C., Dello Russo, A., Picani, C., Palmieri, V., Cameli, S., Corsetti, R., & Pietrangeli, L.

(1995). Echocardiographic size of conductance vessels in athletes and sedentary people. International journal of sports medicine, 16(1), 38–44. https://doi.org/10.1055/s-2007-972961

7. Sugawara, J., Komine, H., Hayashi, K., Yoshizawa, M., Otsuki, T., Shimojo, N., Miyauchi, T., Yokoi, T., Maeda, S., & Tanaka, H. (2007). Systemic alpha-adrenergic and nitric oxide inhibition on basal limb blood flow: effects of endurance training in middle-aged and older adults. American journal of physiology. Heart and circulatory physiology, 293(3), H1466–H1472. https://doi.org/10.1152/ajpheart.00273.2007

8. Brito, A., de Oliveira, C. V., Santos, M., & Santos, A. (2014). High-intensity exercise promotes postexercise hypotension greater than moderate intensity in elderly hypertensive individuals. Clinical physiology and functional imaging, 34(2), 126–132. https://doi.org/10.1111/cpf.12074

9. Nascimento, D., Tibana, R. A., Benik, F. M., Fontana, K. E., Ribeiro Neto, F., Santana, F. S., Santos-Neto, L., Silva, R. A., Silva, A. O., Farias, D. L., Balsamo, S., & Prestes, J. (2014). Sustained effect of resistance training on blood pressure and hand grip strength following a detraining period in elderly hypertensive women: a pilot study. Clinical interventions in aging, 9, 219–225. https://doi.org/10.2147/CIA.S56058

10. Lovell, D. I., Cuneo, R., & Gass, G. C. (2009). Resistance training reduces the blood pressure response of older men during submaximum aerobic exercise. Blood pressure monitoring, 14(4), 137–144. https://doi.org/10.1097/MBP.0b013e32832e0644

11. Vincent, K. R., Vincent, H. K., Braith, R. W., Bhatnagar, V., & Lowenthal, D. T. (2003). Strength training and hemodynamic responses to exercise. The American journal of

geriatric cardiology, 12(2), 97–106. https://doi.org/10.1111/j.1076-7460.2003.01588.x

12. Kelley, G. A., & Kelley, K. S. (2010). Isometric handgrip exercise and resting blood pressure: a meta-analysis of randomized controlled trials. Journal of hypertension, 28(3), 411–418. https://doi.org/10.1097/HJH.0b013e3283357d16

13. Spence, A. L., Carter, H. H., Naylor, L. H., & Green, D. J. (2013). A prospective randomized longitudinal study involving 6 months of endurance or resistance exercise. Conduit artery adaptation in humans. The Journal of physiology, 591(5), 1265–1275. https://doi.org/10.1113/jphysiol.2012.247387

14. Dos Santos, E. S., Asano, R. Y., Filho, I. G., Lopes, N. L., Panelli, P., Nascimento, D., Collier, S. R., & Prestes, J. (2014). Acute and chronic cardiovascular response to 16 weeks of combined eccentric or traditional resistance and aerobic training in elderly hypertensive women: a randomized controlled trial. Journal of strength and conditioning research, 28(11), 3073–3084. https://doi.org/10.1519/JSC.0000000000000537

15. Ash, G. I., Eicher, J. D., & Pescatello, L. S. (2013). The promises and challenges of the use of genomics in the prescription of exercise for hypertension: the 2013 update. Current hypertension reviews, 9(2), 130–147. https://doi.org/10.2174/15734021113099990010

16. Paul D. Thompson, Barry A. Franklin, Gary J. Balady, Steven N. Blair, Domenico Corrado, N.A. Mark EstesIII, Janet E. Fulton, Neil F. Gordon, William L. Haskell, Mark S. Link, Barry J. Maron, Murray A. Mittleman, Antonio Pelliccia, Nanette K. Wenger, Stefan N. Willich, and Fernando Costa , Exercise and Acute Cardiovascular Events Originally published27 Apr

2007https://doi.org/10.1161/CIRCULATIONAHA.107.181485Circulation. 2007;115:2358–2368

17. James E. Sharman, Andre La Gerche, Jeff S. Coombes, Exercise and Cardiovascular Risk in Patients With Hypertension, American Journal of Hypertension, Volume 28, Issue 2, February 2015, Pages 147–158, https://doi.org/10.1093/ajh/hpu191

18. Ried, K., Frank, O.R., Stocks, N.P. et al. Effect of garlic on blood pressure: A systematic review and meta-analysis. BMC Cardiovasc Disord 8, 13 (2008). https://doi.org/10.1186/1471-2261-8-13

19. Iwaniak, A., Minkiewicz, P. and Darewicz, M. (2014), Food-Originating ACE Inhibitors, Including Antihypertensive Peptides, as Preventive Food Components in Blood Pressure Reduction. Comprehensive Reviews in Food Science and Food Safety, 13: 114-134. https://doi.org/10.1111/1541-4337.12051

20. Alexander W. (2014). Hypertension: is it time to replace drugs with nutrition and nutraceuticals?. P & T : a peer-reviewed journal for formulary management, 39(4), 291–295.

21. K T Khaw, E Barrett-Connor, Dietary potassium and blood pressure in a population, The American Journal of Clinical Nutrition, Volume 39, Issue 6, June 1984, Pages 963–968, https://doi.org/10.1093/ajcn/39.6.963

22. Alfonso Siani, Pasquale Strazzullo, Angela Giacco, et al. Increasing the Dietary Potassium Intake Reduces the Need for Antihypertensive Medication. Ann Intern Med.1991;115:753-759. [Epub ahead of print 10 March 2020]. doi:10.7326/0003-4819-115-10-753

23. Bain L.K.M., Myint P.K., Jennings A., Lentjes M.A.H., Luben R.N., Khaw K.-T., Wareham N.J., Welch A.A. The

relationship between dietary magnesium intake, stroke and its major risk factors, blood pressure and cholesterol, in the EPIC-Norfolk cohort (2015) International Journal of Cardiology, 196 , pp. 108-114.

24. Vikas Kapil, Rayomand S. Khambata, Amy Robertson, Mark J. Caulfield, and Amrita Ahluwalia . Dietary Nitrate Provides Sustained Blood Pressure Lowering in Hypertensive Patients. 2014https://doi.org/10.1161/HYPERTENSIONAHA.114.04675Hypertension. 2015;65:320–327

25. Delfin Rodriguez-Leyva, Wendy Weighell, Andrea L. Edel, Renee LaVallee, Elena Dibrov, Reinhold Pinneker, Thane G. Maddaford, Bram Ramjiawan, Michel Aliani, Randolph Guzman, and Grant N. Pierce. Potent Antihypertensive Action of Dietary Flaxseed in Hypertensive Patients. 2013/ https://doi.org/10.1161/HYPERTENSIONAHA.113.02094Hypertension. 2013;62:1081–1089

26. James, Jack E. PhD Critical Review of Dietary Caffeine and Blood Pressure: A Relationship That Should Be Taken More Seriously, Psychosomatic Medicine: January-February 2004 - Volume 66 - Issue 1 - p 63-71 doi: 10.1097/10.PSY.0000107884.78247.F9

27. Nurminen, ML., Niittynen, L., Korpela, R. et al. Coffee, caffeine and blood pressure: a critical review. Eur J Clin Nutr 53, 831–839 (1999). https://doi.org/10.1038/sj.ejcn.1600899

28. Terry R. Hartley, Bong Hee Sung, Gwendolyn A. Pincomb, Thomas L. Whitsett, Michael F. Wilson, and William R. Lovallo. Hypertension Risk Status and Effect of Caffeine on Blood Pressure.

2000https://doi.org/10.1161/01.HYP.36.1.137Hypertension. 2000;36:137–141

29. Arthur Eumann Mesas, Luz M Leon-Muñoz, Fernando Rodriguez-Artalejo, Esther Lopez-Garcia, The effect of coffee on blood pressure and cardiovascular disease in hypertensive individuals: a systematic review and meta-analysis, The American Journal of Clinical Nutrition, Volume 94, Issue 4, October 2011, Pages 1113–1126, https://doi.org/10.3945/ajcn.111.016667

30. Hodgson, Jonathan M.1,2; Puddey, Ian B.1; Burke, Valerie1; Beilin, Lawrence J.1; Jordan, Nerissa1 Effects on blood pressure of drinking green and black tea, Journal of Hypertension: April 1999 - Volume 17 - Issue 4 - p 457-463

31. Onakpoya, E. Spencer, C. Heneghan, M. Thompson,.The effect of green tea on blood pressure and lipid profile: A systematic review and meta-analysis of randomized clinical trials,Nutrition, Metabolism and Cardiovascular Diseases,Volume 24, Issue 8, 2014,Pages 823-836, ISSN 0939-4753, https://doi.org/10.1016/j.numecd.2014.01.016.

32. Greyling A, Ras RT, Zock PL, Lorenz M, Hopman MT, et al. (2014) The Effect of Black Tea on Blood Pressure: A Systematic Review with Meta-Analysis of Randomized Controlled Trials. PLOS ONE 9(7): e103247. https://doi.org/10.1371/journal.pone.0103247

33. Diane L. McKay, C-Y. Oliver Chen, Edward Saltzman, Jeffrey B. Blumberg, Hibiscus Sabdariffa L. Tea (Tisane) Lowers Blood Pressure in Prehypertensive and Mildly Hypertensive Adults, The Journal of Nutrition, Volume 140, Issue 2, February 2010, Pages 298–303, https://doi.org/10.3945/jn.109.115097

34. Puddey, I.B. and Beilin, L.J. (2006), ALCOHOL IS BAD FOR BLOOD PRESSURE. Clinical and Experimental

Pharmacology and Physiology, 33: 847-852. https://doi.org/10.1111/j.1440-1681.2006.04452.x

35. Husain, K., Ansari, R. A., & Ferder, L. (2014). Alcohol-induced hypertension: Mechanism and prevention. World journal of cardiology, 6(5), 245–252. https://doi.org/10.4330/wjc.v6.i5.245

36. Fresco P.C, Graham A.MDoes potassium supplementation lower blood pressure? A meta-analysis of published trials.(1991) Journal of hypertension 1991 9;465-473

37. Jalal Poorolajal,Fatemeh Zeraati,Ali Reza Soltanian,Vida Sheikh,Elham Hooshmand,Akram Maleki. Oral potassium supplementation for management of essential hypertension: A meta-analysis of randomized controlled trials Published: April 18, 2017https://doi.org/10.1371/journal.pone.0174967

38. Kass, L., Weekes, J. & Carpenter, L. Effect of magnesium supplementation on blood pressure: a meta-analysis. Eur J Clin Nutr 66, 411–418 (2012). https://doi.org/10.1038/ejcn.2012..4

39. Reinhart, K. M., Coleman, C. I., Teevan, C., Vachhani, P., & White, C. M. (2008). Effects of Garlic on Blood Pressure in Patients with and Without Systolic Hypertension: A Meta-Analysis. Annals of Pharmacotherapy, 42(12), 1766–1771. https://doi.org/10.1345/aph.1L319

40. https://examine.com/supplements/garlic/#effect-matrix

41. Ashor, Ammar W.a; Lara, Joseb; Siervo, Marioa Medium-term effects of dietary nitrate supplementation on systolic and diastolic blood pressure in adults, Journal of Hypertension: July 2017 - Volume 35 - Issue 7 - p 1353-1359 doi: 10.1097/HJH.0000000000001305

42. Mario Siervo, Jose Lara, Ikponmwonsa Ogbonmwan, John C. Mathers, Inorganic Nitrate and Beetroot Juice Supplementation Reduces Blood Pressure in Adults: A Systematic Review and Meta-Analysis, The Journal of Nutrition, Volume 143, Issue 6, June 2013, Pages 818–826, https://doi.org/10.3945/jn.112.170233

43. Susalit, E., Agus, N., Effendi, I., Tjandrawinata, R. R., Nofiarny, D., Perrinjaquet-Moccetti, T., & Verbruggen, M. (2011). Olive (Olea europaea) leaf extract effective in patients with stage-1 hypertension: comparison with Captopril. Phytomedicine : international journal of phytotherapy and phytopharmacology, 18(4), 251–258. https://doi.org/10.1016/j.phymed.2010.08.016

44. John Zhang, George Oxinos, John H. Maher,The effect of fruit and vegetable powder mix on hypertensive subjects: a pilot study, Journal of Chiropractic Medicine, Volume 8, Issue 3,2009,Pages 101-106, ISSN 1556-3707, https://doi.org/10.1016/j.jcm.2008.09.004.

45. M C Morris, F Sacks, and B Rosner, Does fish oil lower blood pressure? A meta-analysis of controlled trials.1993https://doi.org/10.1161/01.CIR.88.2.523Circulation. 1993;88:523–533

46. Hoshi, T., Wissuwa, B., Tian, Y., Tajima, N., Xu, R., Bauer, M., Heinemann, S. H., & Hou, S. (2013). Omega-3 fatty acids lower blood pressure by directly activating large-conductance Ca^{2+}-dependent K^+ channels. Proceedings of the National Academy of Sciences of the United States of America, 110(12), 4816–4821. https://doi.org/10.1073/pnas.1221997110

47. Rosenfeldt, F., Haas, S., Krum, H. et al. Coenzyme Q10 in the treatment of hypertension: a meta-analysis of the clinical trials. J Hum Hypertens 21, 297–306 (2007). https://doi.org/10.1038/sj.jhh.1002138

48. Rosenfeldt, F., Hilton, D., Pepe, S. and Krum, H. (2003), Systematic review of effect of coenzyme Q10 in physical exercise, hypertension and heart failure. BioFactors, 18: 91-100. https://doi.org/10.1002/biof.5520180211

49. Harm H.H. Feringa, Dayne A. Laskey, Justine E. Dickson, Craig I. Coleman, The Effect of Grape Seed Extract on Cardiovascular Risk Markers: A Meta-Analysis of Randomized Controlled Trials, Journal of the American Dietetic Association, Volume 111, Issue 8, 2011, Pages 1173-1181, ISSN 0002-8223, https://doi.org/10.1016/j.jada.2011.05.015.

50. Zhang, H., Liu, S., Li, L., Liu, S., Liu, S., Mi, J., & Tian, G. (2016). The impact of grape seed extract treatment on blood pressure changes: A meta-analysis of 16 randomized controlled trials. Medicine, 95(33), e4247. https://doi.org/10.1097/MD.0000000000004247

51. Marc P. McRae, High-dose folic acid supplementation effects on endothelial function and blood pressure in hypertensive patients: a meta-analysis of randomized controlled clinical trials, Journal of Chiropractic Medicine, Volume 8, Issue 1, 2009,Pages 15-24,ISSN 1556-3707, https://doi.org/10.1016/j.jcm.2008.09.001.

52. Mirenayat, M.S., Moradi, S., Mohammadi, H. et al. Effect of L-Citrulline Supplementation on Blood Pressure: a Systematic Review and Meta-Analysis of Clinical Trials. Curr Hypertens Rep 20, 98 (2018). https://doi.org/10.1007/s11906-018-0898-3

53. Alexa Cloud, Dwan Vilcins, Bradley McEwen, The effect of hawthorn (Crataegus spp.) on blood pressure: A systematic review, Advances in Integrative Medicine, Volume 7, Issue 3, 2020, Pages 167-175, ISSN 2212-9588, https://doi.org/10.1016/j.aimed.2019.09.002.

54. Aneliya Parvanova, Matias Trillini, Manuel A Podestà, Ilian P Iliev, Carolina Aparicio, Annalisa Perna, Francesco Peraro, Nadia Rubis, Flavio Gaspari, Antonio Cannata, Silvia Ferrari, Antonio C Bossi, Roberto Trevisan, Sreejith Parameswaran, Jonathan S Chávez-Iñiguez, Fahrudin Masnic, Sidy Mohamed Seck, Teerayuth Jiamjariyaporn, Monica Cortinovis, Luca Perico, Kanishka Sharma, Giuseppe Remuzzi, Piero Ruggenenti, David G Warnock, Blood Pressure and Metabolic Effects of Acetyl-L-Carnitine in Type 2 Diabetes: DIABASI Randomized Controlled Trial, Journal of the Endocrine Society, Volume 2, Issue 5, May 2018, Pages 420–436, https://doi.org/10.1210/js.2017-00426

55. Askarpour, M., Hadi, A., Dehghani Kari Bozorg, A. et al. Effects of L-carnitine supplementation on blood pressure: a systematic review and meta-analysis of randomized controlled trials. J Hum Hypertens 33, 725–734 (2019). https://doi.org/10.1038/s41371-019-0248-1

56. Alexandros N. Vgontzas, MD, Duanping Liao, PhD, Edward O. Bixler, PhD, George P. Chrousos, MD, Antonio Vela-Bueno, MD, Insomnia with Objective Short Sleep Duration is Associated with a High Risk for Hypertension, Sleep, Volume 32, Issue 4, April 2009, Pages 491–497, https://doi.org/10.1093/sleep/32.4.491

57. Grandner M, Mullington JM, Hashmi SD, Redeker NS, Watson NF, Morgenthaler TI. Sleep duration and hypertension: analysis of > 700,000 adults by age and sex. J Clin Sleep Med. 2018;14(6):1031–1039

58. Haack, M., Serrador, J., Cohen, D., Simpson, N., Meier-Ewert, H. and Mullington, J.M. (2013), Increasing sleep duration to lower beat-to-beat blood pressure: a pilot study. J Sleep Res, 22: 295-304. https://doi.org/10.1111/jsr.12011.

59. Björn Folkow (2001) Mental Stress and its Importance for Cardiovascular Disorders; Physiological Aspects, "From-Mice-to-Man", Scandinavian Cardiovascular Journal, 35:3, 163-172, DOI: 10.1080/cdv.35.3.163.172

60. B Folkow, "Structural factor" in primary and secondary hypertension,1990https://doi.org/10.1161/01.HYP.16.1.89Hypert ension. 1990;16:89–101

61. Orfeu M. Buxton, Milena Pavlova, Emily W. Reid, Wei Wang, Donald C. Simonson, Gail K. Adler, Sleep Restriction for 1 Week Reduces Insulin Sensitivity in Healthy Men, Diabetes Sep 2010, 59 (9) 2126-2133; DOI: 10.2337/db09-0699

62. Bönner G. Hyperinsulinemia, insulin resistance, and hypertension. Journal of Cardiovascular Pharmacology. 1994 ;24 Suppl 2:S39-49.

63. Christopher John Worsnop , Matthew Thomas Naughton , Colin Edwin Barter , Trefor Owen Morgan , Adrianne Ila Anderson , And Robert J. Pierce, American Journal of Respiratory and Critical Care Medicine Volume 157, Issue 1 The Prevalence of Obstructive Sleep Apnea in Hypertensives https://doi.org/10.1164/ajrccm.157.1.9609063

64. Logan, Alexander G.a,c; Perlikowski, Sandra M.a; Mente, Andrewa; Tisler, Andrasa; Tkacova, Ruzenab; Niroumand, Mitrab; Leung, Richard S. T.b; Bradley, T. Douglasb,c High prevalence of unrecognized sleep apnoea in drug-resistant hypertension, Journal of Hypertension: December 2001 - Volume 19 - Issue 12 - p 2271-2277

65. K. Mae Hla, James B. Skatrud, Laurel Finn, Mari Palta, Terry Young, The Effect of Correction of Sleep-Disordered Breathing on BP in Untreated Hypertension,Chest Volume 122,

Issue 4,2002, Pages 1125-1132, ISSN 0012-3692, https://doi.org/10.1378/chest.122.4.1125.

66. Karolina Janků,Michal Šmotek,Eva Fárková & Jana Kopřivová . Block the light and sleep well: Evening blue light filtration as a part of cognitive behavioral therapy for insomnia Chronobiology International, Volume 37, Issue 2Pages 248-259 |

   a. https://doi.org/10.1080/07420528.2019.1692859

67. Houston M. C. (2011). The importance of potassium in managing hypertension. Current hypertension reports, 13(4), 309–317. https://doi.org/10.1007/s11906-011-0197-8

Other Books by This Author

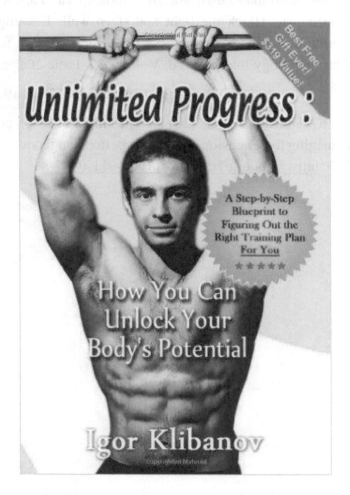

Unlimited Progress: How You Can Unlock Your Body's Potential

Whether you are new to exercise or a competitive athlete, at some point in your training you will hit the **dreaded plateau**. After a period of progression, suddenly you hit a wall. Your weight loss stalls. Your performance stagnates. Your body and your mind are in a rut and you may be tempted to just give up.

While everyone hits a plateau, our bodies are not the same. Generic training programs may work initially but inevitably your body will stop responding in the same way. You have your own unique body, and to identify your greatest opportunities for improvement, you will find lots of **low-tech, high-effectiveness tests** to help you identify which training methods to use.

Chances are you've already tried some different training methods, but you might be frustrated because they haven't worked as well as you'd like. The truth is no matter what your level is, there will always be weaknesses, just because strengthening previous weaknesses and making them into strengths will open up other weaknesses.

The encouraging thing about that is that you can always progress, and by using the diagnostic tests that are covered in the book, you'll **know exactly where to look to make progress**.

But generic programs are not the answer to consistent and continual progress. This book covers tests for 10 different fitness qualities:

- Fat Loss
- Muscle Mass
- Strength
- Power
- Speed
- Muscular Endurance
- Aerobic Endurance

- Anaerobic Endurance

- Flexibility

- Coordination

Filled with flowcharts and illustrative pictures you will understand and be able to easily apply the content to customize a program that works for you. Say good-bye to plateaus as you learn how to reach your ultimate potential. Whether you are a beginner starting a weight loss program, an athlete or a coach who must tailor training programs, this book will teach you to how to work with your body and your unique needs to design a program that will help you keep reaching your goals.

To get a copy of this book, visit **https://amzn.to/2IRB5yR**.

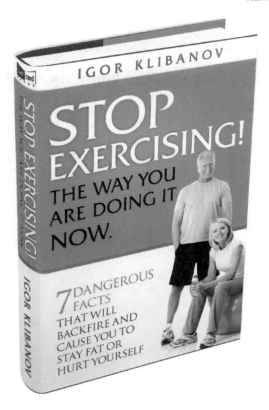

STOP EXERCISING! The Way You Are Doing it Now

Are you trying to lose fat, get toned and have more energy? This book teaches you, step-by-step, how you can lose 10 - 100 pounds or more safely, effectively, and without regaining it. This is done without gimmicks, fancy equipment, questionable supplements or confusion. Based on the methodology we've successfully used with thousands of personal training clients, this book teaches you how to lose fat, get toned and have more energy from the "inside out." By focusing on your body's internal environment, you let fat loss happen as a side effect of getting healthier. And anyone can do this if they just follow the proven, step-by-step instructions in this book.

You will learn how to lose fat by balancing your hormones, reducing stress, improving your digestion, and more.

To grab a copy of this book, visit **https://amzn.to/34j2cec**.

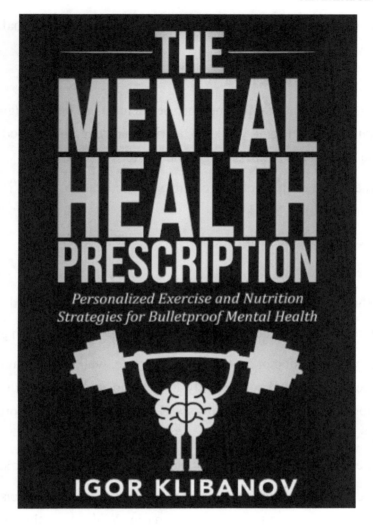

The Mental Health Prescription: Personalized Exercise and Nutrition Strategies for Bulletproof Mental Health

You're probably considering this book because you're struggling with mental health. Maybe it's anxiety, maybe it's depression, PTSD, or something else. Or perhaps, you have friends or family members with these conditions. Or perhaps you're a health/fitness professional, wanting to help your clients or patients.

If so, then this book is for you.

You, your friend, family member or client(s) has been struggling with a mental health issue, and you keep hearing that "exercise is good for you." But you're not really sure exactly what to do.

I mean, when a doctor prescribes a medication, there is a lot of precision behind it. You know:

•The name of the medication.

•The dosage.

•Whether it should be taken with food or without food, and

•Whether it should be taken in the morning, noon or evening

But when the doctor recommends exercise, well, the recommendation is vague. You don't know exactly how to do it. You need the exercise prescription for different conditions. To know the exercise prescription you need to know:

•The type of exercise, such as: cardio, strength training, or stretching

•The frequency: how many days per week you should exercise. It's not always a "more is better" type of scenario. With some things there's a "sweet spot", where too little is not stimulating, and too much is implausible. The "sweet spot" varies condition-by-condition, and person-to-person

•The duration: how long you should exercise for

•The intensity: at what percent of your maximal effort do you exercise?

Just as a doctor does not prescribe the same medication for different conditions, nor does it make sense to do the same exercise for different conditions. What's good for depression may actually make anxiety worse (you might be wondering "I have BOTH anxiety and depression. What do I do???" Don't worry my friend, I won't leave you hanging. That's covered in the chapter on "how to individualize").

What's good for one condition may not be good for another. As a result of using the right exercise and nutrition prescription, you can expect to:

•Reverse your condition(s)•Improved your performance at work

•Be able to focus better

•Start new relationships that are personally satisfying

•Lose weight Get more toned

•Have more energy

•Sleep better

•Achieve mental clarity and a peace of mind

…and lots more.

I've written the book to be as thorough as possible, but I know that with all the details, it can get overwhelming. That's why in the conclusion of this book, you'll find a quick reference guide. No theory, just practice. If you don't want to learn about the physiology behind mental health, and you're more of a "just tell me what to do" kind of person, just flip to the conclusion, and follow the recommendations in there. It will take you less than 5 minutes to get through that.

To grab a copy of this book, visit **https://amzn.to/3jiFl6T**.

Services Offered by the Author

Personal Training and Nutritional Consulting

If you're in or around the Greater Toronto Area, you can see whether you qualify to train with the author, or one of his team members.

The training starts with an initial assessment, where the author learns about you and your goals, injuries, medical conditions, medications, and more.

After the initial assessment, the author crafts an exercise and nutrition program made to fit you like a finely-tailored suit.

As you continue making progress, adjustments will be made to your program, to make sure you're moving closer and closer to your goal.

If you'd like to see whether this is right for you, simply email Igor@TorontoFitnessOnline.com.

Online Coaching

If you're outside the Greater Toronto Area, but want to benefit from professional expertise, the author has specifically trained a hand-picked, elite team of fitness professionals to train clients remotely.

The online coaching starts with an initial assessment, where your coach learns about you and your goals, injuries, medical conditions, medications, and more.

After that, an exercise and/or nutrition program will be crafted to fit your goals, your body, your time and equipment availability.

Adjustments to the program will be made on a regular basis, to keep you progressing.

If you'd like to see whether this is right for you, simply email Igor@TorontoFitnessOnline.com.

Consulting

If you don't need a program made for you, but you just have questions to ask, and you're confused by all the information out there, so you just want the highest-quality, most accurate information handed to you on a silver platter, we can do that.

You'll save tons of time and frustration on the research and trial and error it takes to figure out what works for you.

If you'd like to see whether this is right for you, simply email Igor@TorontoFitnessOnline.com.

Public Speaking

Igor Klibanov is one of the most sought-after wellness speakers in the Greater Toronto Area, having delivered over 400 speaking engagements (at the time of this writing) to some of Canada's largest corporations, including the Royal Bank of Canada, IBM, Bosch, and many others.

Topics include:

1. STOP EXERCISING! The Way You Are Doing it Now

2. Exercise and Nutrition for Mental Health

3. 8 Hidden Reasons You Can't Lose Weight

4. Everything You Wanted to Know About Nutritional

Supplements, But Were Afraid to Ask

5. No Pain, All Gain: How to Exercise the Right Way For YOUR Chronic Condition

6. Exercise for Different Body Types

7. Fitness for Females

8. Weight Loss for Women Over 40

9. Healthy Food That Poisons: Why You're Getting Sicker and Fatter Despite Eating Healthier

10. How to Get a Flat Stomach, Round Butt and Lose Weight

11. How to Prevent Neck Pain and Lower Back Pain

12. Running for Non-Runners

13. Stand Up Straight. A 4-Step Approach to Fixing Your Posture

14. How to Double Your Testosterone Naturally in 6 Months

15. How to lose 10, 20, 50 or more pounds without crash dieting

16. Stress Management for the Busy Professional

17. How to Change Your Mind to Change Your Body

18. Fitness over 50

19. A New Model of Pain

20. Workshop: Exercise progressions and Regressions

21. Workshop: Self tissue release

To book Igor for a speaking engagement, email Igor@TorontoFitnessOnline.com.

Made in United States
Troutdale, OR
11/28/2023

14960501R00080